Neuroscie ‖‖ ‖ ‖‖‖‖‖‖‖‖‖‖‖‖‖‖‖‖‖‖‖‖‖‖‖‖ ‖ ‖‖‖ ‖‖

Frencha✔ KU-669-739

Demos Medical Publishing, Inc., 386 Park Avenue South, New York, New York 10016

©**Academic Information Systems, 1999**

Prescribing information, dosing, side-effects and adverse reactions described in this book may change. The reader should carefully review package insert information prior to prescribing any of the medications referenced.

Any errors, omissions or copyright infringements are unintentional. The publisher will be pleased to make any necessary arrangements if they have inadvertently missed any previous copyrights.

Printed in the United States of America

Use of botulinum toxin type A in pain management: a clinician's guide

---

- Practical, easy-to-read introduction to an emerging treatment for painful syndromes associated with involuntary muscle contraction
- Key facts about botulinum toxin type A
- Overview of myofascial pain syndromes
- Trigger point injections: evidence in the literature
- Treatment of painful spasticity and dystonia
- Equipment and injection techniques
- Sample documentation templates
- Coding and reimbursement for pain and botulinum toxin type A
- Seminar and workshop information

Use of Botulinum Toxin Type A in Pain Management: a clinician's guide

Martin K. Childers, D.O.
Assistant Professor
Department of Physical Medicine and Rehabilitation
University of Missouri-Columbia
Columbia, Missouri

Daniel J. Wilson, PhD
Assistant Professor
Department of Physical Medicine and Rehabilitation
University of Missouri-Columbia
Columbia, Missouri

Diane Simison, PhD
Principal
Epinomics Research, Inc
Arlington, Virginia

Illustrations by:
Kari C. Childers
Columbia, Missouri

Contents

C20 45025 1

Foreword

The art of life is the art of avoiding pain; and he is the best pilot, who steers clearest of the rocks and shoals with which it is beset.
---Thomas Jefferson

It is the beauty of medical science that a substance such as botulinum toxin has been harnessed to accomplish therapeutic purposes. Feared as a cause of death from paralysis, I am sure that it would seem unlikely to the man on the street that any good could come from this toxic substance. Nonetheless, the use of minute amounts of the purified toxin has become more commonplace in medical practice.

This little gem of a book by Drs Childers, Wilson and Simison will undoubtedly aid the practitioner learn the practice of pain relief and restoration of function through the judicious use of botulinum toxin. By following the clear instructions and informative illustrations, practitioners will become familiar with the basic knowledge and skills needed to harness this important clinical technique. Only through careful study of the principles and application of the techniques described herein can we practice effective (and cost-effective) medical care in this emerging area.

Steve M. Gnatz, MD, MHA
Professor and Chair
Department of Physical Medicine and Rehabilitation
University of Missouri-Columbia
Columbia, Missouri

Preface

Treatment of painful syndromes of muscle remains incompletely understood and controversial. While the use of botulinum toxin type A (BTX-A) in the treatment of conditions associated with involuntary muscle contraction, such as focal dystonia and spasticity, is supported by prospective, randomized clinical research, comparable research in pain syndromes remains to be fully explored. Accordingly, therapy with botulinum toxin type A for such "off-label" use should be carefully considered. The purpose of this introductory guide is to provide both general direction and practical details for the busy clinician. The anatomic drawings for injection localization and accompanying dosing information are intended only as general guidelines; therapy with botulinum toxin type A must always be individualized not only for the patient's needs, but also for the clinician's expertise. This handbook should be used as a convenient reference source and not as a substitute for clinical training in the use of botulinum toxin.

Martin K. Childers, D.O.

1
CHAPTER

Introduction

This handbook will outline potential uses of botulinum toxin type A (BOTOX®) for pain management. Although the FDA licensed uses for botulinum toxin type A do not address pain management, this product currently is being used by a range of medical specialists to address pain control of various etiologies. However, there is insufficient available information that directly addresses clinical guidelines or provides the necessary knowledge base to most appropriately use botulinum toxin type A (BTX-A) for pain management. The purpose of this handbook therefore, is to provide some clinical guidance to physicians regarding the use of BTX-A, based upon similar applications in a variety of neuromuscular disorders.

The text highlights essential features one should know about BTX-A before treating patients for pain, and additional sources of information are listed at the end of the text in Appendix A.

TOPICS

- Mechanism of action (MOA)[1]
- Concept of LD50
- Dosing and administration [2]
- Basic muscle physiology
- Treatment(s) which might be helpful in conjunction

with BTX-A therapy
• Contraindications

APPLICATIONS

In 1989, the Food and Drug Administration (FDA) licensed botulinum toxin type A (BOTOX®) in the US for treatment of the following in patients over the age of 12 years:

• strabismus (a condition in which one or both eyes do not move together in tandem)
• essential blepharospasm (involuntary blinking)
• hemifacial spasm (involuntary facial muscle spasms)[3]

But in addition to the approved uses in the US, there are other published uses of BTX-A, which include:

achalasia	myofascial pain syndrome
anismus	
cervical dystonia	occupational dystonia
detrussor-sphincter	pain (muscle spasm)
dysinergia	piriformis muscle syndrome
essential blepharospasm	
essential tremor	spasmotic dysphonia
facial wrinkles	spasticity
hemifacial spasm	strabismus
hyperhydrosis	

Beyond publications, noteworthy medical organizations have commented on the effectiveness and safety of

BTX-A. The National Institutes of Health Consensus Development Conference published a statement in 1990[2] which summarized the indications and contraindications of BTX-A usage for the treatment of a variety of conditions. The NIH conference endorsed the use of BTX-A as safe and effective for the symptomatic treatment of adductor spasmodic dysphonia, blepharospasm, cervical dystonia, hemifacial spasm, jaw-closing oromandibular dystonia and strabismus. The same year, the Therapeutics and Technology Assessment Subcommittee of the American Academy of Neurology further endorsed the use of BTX-A for the symptomatic treatment of these conditions.[4]

While the use of EMG for injection localization of BTX-A in pain management might improve clinical response, relevant information on EMG usage is contained in Chapter 7 for those readers not familiar with this tool. Overall, previous experience with EMG is not necessary.

EMG Considerations:

- EMG can be helpful, but not mandatory
- EMG used for injection localization is a much simpler process than for diagnostic purposes.
- EMG does require working knowledge of functional anatomy and neuromuscular physiology, but relevant information is offered throughout this text.

REFERENCES

1. Coffield JA, Considine RB, Simpson LL. The site and mechanism of action of botulinum neurotoxin. In: Jankovic J, Hallett M, eds. Therapy with botulinum toxin. New York: Marcel Dekker, Inc., 1994:3-14.
2. Anonymous. Consensus conference. Clinical uses of botulinum toxin. National Institutes of Health. [Review] [0 refs]. Connecticut Medicine 1991;55:471-477.

3. Jankovic J, Brin MF. Therapeutic uses of botulinum toxin. [Review]. NEJM 1991;324:1186-1194.
4. Anonymous. Training guidelines for the use of botulinum toxin for the treatment of neurologic disorders. Report of the Therapeutics and Technology Assessment Subcommittee of the American Academy of Neurology. Neurology 1994;44:2401-2403.

2
CHAPTER

Key Facts

Botulinum toxin, produced by the anaerobic bacteria, *Clostridium botulinum*, is a rod shaped, gram positive organism found in soil and water. BTX-A is composed of a family of neurotoxins (designated as types A, B, C1, C2, D, E, F, and G) which have similar properties.[1-3] BTX-A causes degrees of flaccid (rather than rigid, or tetanic) paralysis by blocking acetylcholine (required for muscle contraction) from release at the nerve terminal. Therefore, therapeutic benefit may be obtained by exploiting pharmacologic properties of carefully administered regional application of this purified neurotoxin.[4; 5]

Botulinum toxin's putative success in pain management is central to its ability to block acetylcholine from being released at the synapse. Another important fact is that BTX-A only acts upon motor nerve endings and does not effect sensory nerve fibers.[6] These topics are explored in greater detail in Chapter 3.

However, before considering the physiology of BTX-A in greater detail, let us first consider some general information.

MEDIAN LETHAL DOSE

Botulinum toxin's median lethal dose (LD50) has been determined across several animal species, but not experimentally determined in humans.

A unit of BTX-A is usually defined in terms of its biological potency. One (mouse) unit (MU) of BTX-A equals the LD50 for a 20 gm Swiss-Webster mouse.[1, 2 ,7] Yet, BTX-A sensitivity has been found to vary among different species. The LD50 in monkeys has been determined to be 39 U/kg. Based on these findings from primate studies, a human LD50 is estimated to be approximately 3000 units for a 70kg adult. Typical doses for larger muscle groups range from about 60 to 400 total units given in a single treatment.

However, due to an inadequate understanding of the complete dose response curve in humans, a relative ceiling dose of 360 units given no sooner than 12 weeks apart is recommended. [8,9]

SIDE EFFECTS

Since the mechanism of action of BTX-A is so specific, side effects are uncommon and systemic effects rare. A flu-like syndrome has been reported, but is generally short-lived.[5] Other side-effects have been reported, but are not necessarily a result of BTX-A treatment. They include muscle soreness, headaches, light-headedness, fever, chills, hypertension, weakness, diarrhea and abdominal pain.

Muscular weakness, the predominant effect of BTX-A injection, also may be considered a negative side effect when weakness occurs in an undesired area, or when weakness is greater than intended. Therefore, patients should be informed of the potential for either too much weakness in the area injected or in nearby muscles.

It is important that clinicians understand the functional consequences of unintended weakness. While over-weakening the muscles that curl the toes may have little, if any, undesirable consequences, spread of toxin into the muscles that control swallowing (which can occur when injecting muscles near the larynx, such as the proximal part of the sternocleidomastoid muscle) may result in difficulty swallowing.[10,11] While clinicians should be generally cautious of this potential negative side effect of botulinum toxin, the following details area of particular consideration:

Use Caution When Injecting These Muscles

- **Extensors of the knee joint (quadraceps)**
  Since the knee extensors help maintain the center of gravity in front of the knee, weakening these muscles may result in a shift in center of gravity behind the knee during walking. This may increase energy required for walking or standing, or even worse, produce an inability to walk.

- **Ankle extensors**
  The tibialis anterior muscle is important in clearing the toe during normal walking. Weakening this ankle extensor too much can cause a patient to drag the toes during the swing phase of gait.

- **Neck extensors**
  Although the cervical paraspinal muscles may be a common source of painful spasms in a variety of conditions, weakening this muscle group can produce head drooping during activities like

6

driving, reading, or working at a computer terminal.

- **Anterior neck muscles**

  Dysphagia may result from diffusion of toxin into nearby muscles of the pharynx. Special precaution should be used when injecting the SCM, scalenes, or other structures of the anterior neck. Dysphagia, when it occurs, is often transient, occurring within approximately one week of injection and lasting about two weeks. Most patients can be managed with a soft diet for a few days. Referral to speech pathology for video fluoroscopy may be warranted if there concern for aspiration.

Relative Contraindications

- Conditions of generalized muscular weakness such as neuromuscular disorders, systemic illness, progressive myopathies.
- Patient is hesitant or does not fully understand risks/benefits
- Profound atrophy of the target muscle(s)
- Aminoglycoside antibiotic therapy (BTX-A may potentiate general weakness.

REFERENCES

1. Coffield JA, Considine RB, Simpson LL. The site and mechanism of action of botulinum neurotoxin. In: Jankovic J, Hallett M, eds. Therapy with botulinum toxin. New York: Marcel Dekker, Inc., 1994:3-14.
2. Mellanby J. Comparative activities of tetanus and botulinum toxins [Review]. Neuroscience 1084;11:29-34.
3. Melling J, Hambleton P, Shone CC. Clostridium botulinum toxins: nature and preparation for clinical use. Eye 1988;2:16-23.
4. Anonymous. Consensus conference. Clinical use of botulinum toxin. National Institutes of Health. [Review] [0 refs]. Connecticut Medicine

1991;55:471-477.
5. Jankovic J, Brin MF. Therapeutic uses of botulinum toxin. [Review]. NEJM 1991;324:1186-1194.
6. Sellin L. The action of botulinum toxin at the neuromuscular junction [Review]. Med Biol 1981;59:11-20.
7. de Paiva A, Ashton A, Foran P, Schiavo G, Montecucco C, Dolly J. Botulinum A like type B and tetanus toxins fulfills criteria for being a zinc-dependent protease. J Neurochem 1993;61:2338-2341.
8. Spasticity: Etiology, Evaluation, Management, and the Role of Botulinum Toxin Type A, MF Brin, editor. Muscle Nerve 1997;20(suppl 6):S208-S220.
9. Greene P, Fahn S: Development of Antibodies to Botulinum Toxin Type A in Patients with Torticollis Treated with Injections of Botulinum toxin Type A, in DasGupta BR (ed): Botulinum and Tetanus Neurotoxins: Neurotransmission and Biomedical Aspects. New York, Plenum Press, 1993: pp 651-654.
10. Jankovic J, Schwartz K, Donovan DT. Botulinum toxin treatment of cranial-cervical dystonia, spasmodic dysphonia, other focal dystonias and hemifacial spasm. J Neurol Neurosurg Psychiatry 1990;53:633-639.
11. Lorentz IT, Subramaniam SS, Yiannikas C. Treatment of idiopathic spasmodic torticollis with botulinum-A toxin: a pilot study of 19 patients. Medical Journal of Australia 1990;152:528-530.

3

CHAPTER

Neuromuscular physiology for botulinum toxin type A users

KEY FACTS
- Acetylcholine has broad functions as a neurotransmitter throughout the peripheral nervous system
- Botulinum toxin type A blocks the release of acetylcholine
- Physicians can exploit the unique physiological actions of acetylcholine blockade using botulinum toxin type A.
- Understanding how and where acetylcholine functions in the body is key

---

PHYSIOLOGY OF ACETYLCHOLINE (ACh)

ACh in Muscular Contraction

Acetylcholine (figure 3-1) is the major neurotransmitter involved in skeletal muscle contraction. The action of acetylcholine (ACh) in skeletal muscle occurs at the neuromuscular junction. ACh enters the synapse at this junction through its calcium-activated release from the pre-synaptic membrane. It then binds to nicotinic receptors on the postsynaptic muscle membrane. These nicotinic receptors, a type of ionotropic receptor, allow transport of sodium and potassium ions across the post-synaptic cell membrane when activated by ACh. The entry of sodium causes depolarization of the cell membrane and generation of an endplate potential. The endplate potential initiates propagation of an action potential along the cell membrane of the skeletal muscle cell and ultimately skeletal muscle contraction.

BTX-A prevents pre-synaptic ACh release by modulating a membrane bound protein, SNAP 25, which results in the inhibition of the calcium activated release of ACh. Other serotypes of the botulinum toxins (serotypes are designated A-F) act on different neuronal proteins, such as syntaxin or vesicle-associated membrane protein (VAMP).

Acetylcholine Relaxes Smooth Muscle in Some Tissues

In some types of smooth muscle which line the interior of blood vessels (arterioles of some tissue), acetylcholine may cause smooth muscle relaxation. When ACh binds to muscarinic receptors found on blood vessel endothelial cells, the resulting increase in intracellular calcium produces relaxation. (Note that calcium is increased in the endothelial cells, not the smooth muscle cell.) Muscarinic receptors are considered metabatropic, since they act by metabolic pathways involving phospholipases. Calcium acts as a second messenger, triggering the release of a nitric oxide (NO) that diffuses out of the endothelial cell and into the smooth muscle surrounding the blood vessels. The effect of NO is to relax smooth muscle

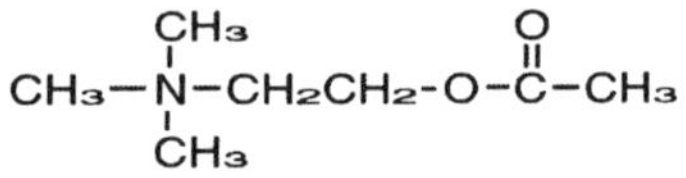

$$CH_3-\overset{\overset{\displaystyle CH_3}{\displaystyle |}}{\underset{\underset{\displaystyle CH_3}{\displaystyle |}}{N}}-CH_2CH_2-O-\overset{\overset{\displaystyle O}{\displaystyle ||}}{C}-CH_3$$

Acetylcholine

Figure 3-1. Chemical structure of acetylcholine (ACh)

Acetylcholine Contracts Smooth Muscle in Other Tissues

Paradoxically, when ACh binds onto other kinds of smooth muscle cell receptors, such as found in the GI tract or around the urinary bladder detrussor, muscle contraction results. When ACh binds to muscarinic receptors in these smooth muscle cells, it increases intracellular calcium and produces contraction. Calcium acts together with calmodulin to add a high-energy phosphate bond onto myosin, a muscle protein. Phosphorylation of myosin triggers an interaction of myosin with actin resulting in muscle contraction.

Acetylcholine Has Other Functions in the Peripheral Nervous System.

Similar to ACh's action at the skeletal muscle nicotinic receptor, the action of ACh binding onto nicotinic receptors in preganglionic sympathetic synapses results in the opening of membrane pores. Opening pores in the preganglionic synapse of the sympathetic system also allows passage of sodium and potassium ions through the cell membrane. Passage of sodium, in particular, depolarizes the postsynaptic nerve cell, and generates an action potential.

How Botulinum Toxin Type A Might Be Used at Preganglionic Sympathetic Synapses

11

Clinicians might exploit the properties of BTX-A in the sympathetic system (at the preganglionic synapse) to alleviate conditions such as sympathetically mediated pain syndromes.

Reflex sympathetic dystrophy (RSD) of the upper limb might be one such example of a condition that might respond to blocking ACh at the preganglionic sympathetic synapse. If the portion of the stellate ganglion (figure 3-2) of the sympathetic chain that innervates the upper limb could be safely localized, and the clinical response with the injection of a short-acting anticholinergic agent (like atracurium) was tested, injection of a very small amount of BTX-A might prove beneficial. The advantage to such treatment would be a longer duration of action than "stellate ganglion blocks" done with sodium channel blockers and steroids. The potential risks would be those associated with blocking any tonic actions of the cervical sympathetic ganglia on viscera that it innervates. However, since the predominate tonic autonomic influence on the heart is parasympathetic, it seems unlikely that removal of any tonic sympathetic influence would be undesirable. Research in animal models might further elucidate any potential side effects of BTX-A in such a setting.

Role of Acetylcholine in Preganglionic Parasympathetic Nerve Transmission

Similar to its action in the sympathetic system, ACh is the major neurotransmitter involved in preganglionic parasympathetic synapses. ACh acts on nicotinic (ionotropic) receptors to open membrane pores, thereby allowing passage of sodium and potassium ions. It is the passage of these ions that recapitulate the action potential originating in the preganglionic nerve.

Uses of Botulinum Toxin Type A at Preganglionic Parasympathetic Synapses

Clinicians might also exploit properties of BTX-A at preganglionic parasympathetic synapses. In fact, one such clinical report (Sherman et al, 1995), investigated injection of BTX-A into the celiac plexus (figure 3-2), a parasympathetic preganglionic region that innervates much of the GI tract, including the pancreas. The hypothesis was that inhibition of autonomic stimulation would decrease the pain of chronic pancreatitis. While the results of this small study were mixed, the rationale for application of agents that block the action of ACh in this setting appears to be reasonable. Other painful conditions associated with overactivity of the parasympathetic nervous system might be amenable to local treatment with BTX-A. Further clinical research is needed in this area to fully explore these possibilities.

Role of Acetylcholine in Postganglionic Parasympathetic Nerve Transmission

Again, ACh is the major neurotransmitter involved in parasympathetic nerve transmission at the postganglionic synapse. Recall that in the parasympathetic system, the postganglionic nerve is relatively short, compared to the longer preganglionic nerve. In smooth muscle tissue innervated by parasympathetic nerve endings, ACh acts on muscarinic (metabatropic) receptors to increase the concentration of intracellular calcium activating the contractile system of smooth muscle.

How Botulinum Toxin Type A Might Be Used at Postganglionic Parasympathetic Synapses

Clinicians can exploit the physiology of ACh at the postganglionic parasympathetic synapses by blocking ACh release at the target origin. One such example is seen in a condition of excessive secretion by the sweat glands, known as hyperhydrosis. For some unfortunate individuals, this excessive sweating about the axilla or palms can result in embarrassing or disabling conditions. Subcutaneous injection of 25-50 MU of BTX-A into the axillary area can alleviate hyperhydrosis for weeks or months.

In some patients, such as children with cerebral palsy, excessive salivation is a considerable problem for caretakers. Excessive salivation is caused by dysregulation of parasympathetic outflow to the salivary glands, which normally produce their own weight in saliva each minute. Since the rate of saliva production is proportional to the blood flow to the glands (regulated by the parasympathetic system), decreasing blood flow should decrease saliva production. Yet, systemic treatment with anticholinergic medications often results in drowsiness, constipation and other undesirable side effects.

However, BTX-A may offer positive response without negative, systemic side effects. Submandibular injections of 5-10 MU BTX-A for involuntary oral-lingual movements may result in diminished outflow of saliva. This is a desirable side effect in many instances, since these individuals also have excessive salivation. Further research would be helpful to more fully investigate the effectiveness of BTX-A treatment for conditions of excessive saliva secretions.

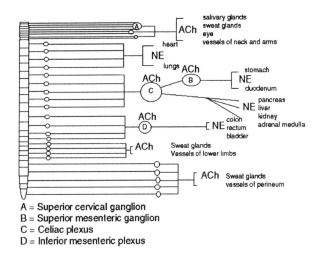

A = Superior cervical ganglion
B = Superior mesenteric ganglion
C = Celiac plexus
D = Inferior mesenteric plexus

Figure 3-2. The autonomic nervous system.

Botulinum Toxin Does Not Block Action Potentials In Sensory Nerves

The primary ions (sodium and potassium) involved in transmission of an action potential in a sensory nerve do not involve acetylcholine. Thus, BTX-A does not affect sensory nerve action potentials. Clinicians may take advantage of this property of BTX-A. For example, in painful foot conditions associated with "alpha rigidity," a type of involuntary muscle contraction of muscles of the

15

calf (sometimes called dystonia or spasticity), physicians may inject the tibial nerve with phenol in order to decrease the nerve supply to the offending muscles. A disadvantage to "phenol neurolysis" is that phenol effects both the sensory and motor nerves. The patient may risk losing sensation to the area supplied by the sensory nerve, or even develop painful dysesthesias in the area supplied by the sensory nerve. BTX-A offers the advantage of being selective for ACh alone, thus sparing any sensory nerve involvement.

Botulinum Toxin Type A May Be More Effective in Slow Twitch Compared to Fast Twitch Muscle

Recall that slow twitch (type I) muscle differs fundamentally from fast twitch (type II) muscle in both structure and function. Type I muscle derives energy from ATP in a molecular pathway that uses oxygen as an important source of electrons. These electrons are used to create high-energy chemical bonds between phosphate and adenosine. This process of oxidative phosphorylation (adding phosphate to adenosine to create ATP) involves myoglobin, an oxygen carrier in muscle cells that impart a dark red color to type I muscle. Alternatively, type II muscle derives energy from ATP using glycolysis, a pathway that does not require oxygen (or myoglobin). Thus, type II muscle is lighter in color than type I muscle.

Botulinum toxin type A seems to be more effective in weakening slow twitch, type I, muscle fibers when compared to type II muscle fibers. This observation might be clinically useful when injecting BTX-A into muscles of the leg, such as the gastroc-soleus complex. Not only is the soleus muscle primarily composed of type I muscle fibers, but an food animal researcher made an interesting observation that muscle lying "closer to the bone" appears to have a greater number of type I fibers when compared to muscle not so "close to the bone." This may be due to the way muscle fibers are used in posture and support. This observation has led the author to target injections of BTX-A into regions of postural muscles that lie closer to the bone whenever possible. Further research in animal models may clarify the clinical usefulness of this curious observation.

In summary, acetylcholine has broad functions as a neurotransmitter throughout the body. Understanding how and where ACh functions in both the autonomic nervous system and in skeletal muscle is important to clinicians who wish to exploit the unique action of BTX-A on ACh blockade. While the pharmacologic action of BTX-A is specific, the broad function of ACh in autonomic ganglia and nicotinic receptors in skeletal muscle allow for a wide potential of clinical applications.

Clinical examples of how BTX-A could be used may be seen in reflex sympathetic dystrophy, chronic pancreatitis, hyperhydrosis, excessive salivation, dystonia, and spasticity. Additionally, targeting injections of BTX-A towards postural muscles lying "closer to the bone" might be beneficial.

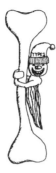

Figure 3-3. BTX-A may be more effective in muscle "closer to the bone".

CHAPTER GLOSSARY

Acetylcholine - a neurotransmitter found in both the central and peripheral nervous system. The term, "cholinergic" refers to agents that have similar systemic actions of acetylcholine. The acronym, SLUD, describes some cholinergic properties: Salivation, Lacrimation, Urination, and Defecation.

Alpha motor neuron – located in the ventral horn of the spinal cord, and innervates extrafusal skeletal muscle fibers. Alpha motor neurons, when improperly activated, may result in alpha rigidity due to disconnections between the cortex and one or more extrapyramidal tracts.

Endplate potential (EPP) – a transient potential on the postjunctional muscle membrane due to ion currents (from

18

sodium and potassium) caused from the binding of ACh to the ionotropic (nicotinic) receptor on the muscle membrane. EPPs can be recorded using electromyography, and the precise location of the neuromuscular junction can be found. This information can help clinicians localize areas for BTX-A injections in some circumstances.

Glycolysis – process of breaking down glucose (a six carbon sugar) into three carbon structures (like pyruvate) creating high-energy intermediates (like ATP). Unlike oxidative phosphorylation, glycolysis does not require oxygen. Used by Type II, fast-twitch muscle cells.

Ionotropic receptor – a membrane "pore" that opens directly upon ligand binding with a receptor allowing passage of ions. The nicotinic receptor, which binds acetylcholine, is a type of ionotropic receptor.

Membrane-associated proteins – many kinds of proteins are found in cell membranes, each with varying functions. One such protein, SNAP-25, is degraded by BTX-A and thereby interferes with calcium-activated release of ACh from the nerve terminal. Other serotypes of the botulinum toxins (serotypes are designated A-F) act on different neuronal proteins, such as syntaxin or vesicle-associated membrane protein (VAMP).

Muscarinic receptor – one of two types of acetylcholine receptors found in various smooth muscle and autonomic synapses throughout the body. Muscarinic receptors are blocked by atropine.

Neuromuscular junction – area between the nerve ending and receptor for acetylcholine. Usually found at the midpoint of each skeletal muscle fiber innervated. The

19

collection of neuromuscular junctions makes up specific patterns in skeletal muscles, some simple while others are complex.

Neurotransmitter - some experts define a neurotransmitter as a substance with the following properties: substance is made within the neuron; activated by a calcium-dependent pathway; effects should be mimicked by exogenous application of the substance while blockade of receptors should abolish these effects; substance must be inactivated by metabolism or reuptake.

Nicotinic receptor is the other type of acetylcholine receptor. These receptors (nicotinic and muscarinic) are named because of their responses to plant alkaloids, muscarine and nicotine. Nicotinic receptors are found in skeletal muscle and at preganglionic sympathetic synapses, preganglionic parasympathetic synapses. Nicotinic receptors are blocked by curare.

Nitric oxide (NO) – a highly permeable gas that acts like a neurotransmitter at synapses between inhibitory motor neurons and some smooth muscle cells. The enzyme NO synthase catalyzes the reaction arginine oxidation into citrulline and NO. NO synthase is stimulated by increased calcium ion inside an endothelial cell. The action of NO in smooth muscle is to relax the muscle.

Oxidative phosphorylation – the biochemical pathway responsible for adding high-energy phosphate bonds to adenosine (creating ATP) and producing CO_2 while consuming molecular oxygen. (See TCA cycle in a chemistry text for a review of the chemistry). Used by Type I, slow-twitch muscle cells.

Peripheral nervous system – everything outside of the central nervous system (brain and spinal cord). The peripheral nervous system is made up of the voluntary or somatic nervous system, which controls motor function, and the involuntary or autonomic nervous system, which controls visceral function (like blood pressure).

Postganglionic – refers to the synapse after the ganglia in either the sympathetic or parasympathetic system. In the parasympathetic outflow, the postganglionic synapse is close to the target tissue. ACh acts on postganglionic muscarinic receptors in the parasympathetic system.

Preganglionic – refers to the synapse just prior to the first ganglia in the sympathetic or parasympathetic outflow. In the sympathetic system, the ACh receptor is a nicotinic receptor.

Skeletal muscle – muscle attached to the body skeleton. Activation of skeletal muscle usually moves or stabilizes a joint.

Smooth muscle – muscle that lines hollow organs or vessels. When smooth muscle contracts, it generally has a propulsive effect or constrictive effect on its tissue.

REFERENCES

- Jacobson, G.R.; Zubay GL: Neurotransmission . In, Biochemistry, Zubay, G.L. (ed.),Wm. C. Brown, Dubuque, IA, 1998.
- Murphy, R.A: Muscle. In, Physiology, fourth edition, Berne,R.M.; Levy, M.N. (ed.), Mosby, St. Louis, 1998.
- Coffield, J.A.; Considine, R.V.; Simpson, L.L.: The site and mechanism of action of botulinum neurotoxin. In, Therapy with botulinum toxin, Jankovic, J.; Hallett, M. (ed.), Marcel Dekker, Inc., New York, 1994.

4
CHAPTER

Overview of the Literature

While many of the chapters refer to specific citations in the literature relevant to information being discussed, this chapter provides a broader look at clinical use of BTX-A in the literature.

A summary of a MEDLINE search for the headings "botulinum toxin," "myofascial pain" and "pain" performed for the period 1966 to September 1997 resulted in 18 references which included 463 subjects, of which 7 studies included "pain" or "myofascial pain" within the article title.[1-18]

The remaining references reported pain response within the context of treatment for underlying spasticity, cervical dystonia, fibromyalgia, focal dystonia and hemifacial spasm, masseteric hypertrophy, painful dystonia in Parkinson's disease, pain of chronic pancreatitis, and writer's cramp. Variables in these studies include dosing, concentration and injection techniques, use of concurrent therapeutic modalities, varying diagnoses, and chronicity of neurologic dysfunction.

Some patients treated for disorders of involuntary muscle contraction (like dystonia) also reported benefits in pain reduction in muscles injected with botulinum toxin.

Table 1. Summary of references generated by MEDLINE search of "botulinum toxin", "myofascial pain" and "pain" for the period 1966 to September 1997.

Reference	N	Diagnosis	Pain Outcome Measures	Mean Dose of BTX-A	Results/Conclusions
Odergren 1994	20	CD	VAS	149 units	VAS ($p<0.01$)
Greene 1990	55	CD	Numeric	118 units	"statistically significant improvement in pain" ($p=.003$)
Jedynak 1990	36	CD	Descriptive	varied	" 20 of 22 positive results… duration over 4 weeks" (French trans.)
Gelb 1989	20	CD	Numeric	varied	16 of 20 patients pain
Tsui 1987	56	CD	Numeric	50-70 units	pain scores 2.1 to 0.9 ($p<0.001$)

23

Reference	N	Diagnosis	Pain Outcome Measures	Mean Dose of BTX-A	Results/Conclusions
Paulson 1996	5	Fibromyalgia	Descriptive	100 units	"Ineffective for pain"
Sherman 1995	7	Chronic pancreatitis	Descriptive	1.5-2.5 U/kg	"Ineffective for pain"
Sheean 1995	2	Writer's cramp	Descriptive	varied	Occurrence of shoulder pain in 2
Pacchetti 1995	30	Parkinson's foot dystonia	McGill pain questionaire	80 units	Improved in all ($p = 0.001$)
Cheshire 1994	6	Myofascial pain	VAS, descriptive	50 units	VAS and most pain descriptors weeks 2-4 ($p<0.05$)
Pierson 1996	39	spasticity	not specified	180 units	improvement in 10 of 13
Monsivais 1996	68	thoracic outlet syndrome	VAS	not specified	VAS ($p = 0.011$)

Reference	N	Diagnosis	Pain Outcome Measures	Mean Dose of BTX-A	Results/Conclusions
Brin 1988	97	focal dystonia and hemifacial spasm	not specified	varied	moderate/marked benefit in 16 of 19 specified
Acquadro 1994	2	myofascial pain	descriptive	50, 150 units	Improved
Girdler 1994	1	facial pain in temporo-mandibular joint (TMJ) dysfunction	descriptive	250 units (Dysport®)	Improved
Girdler 1997	1	chronic muscle spasm of facial arthromyalgia	descriptive	250 units (Dysport®)	"48 h later ... complete cessation of facial pain"
Moore 1994	1	masseteric hypertrophy	NA	100	NA

REPORTED EFFICACY FOR PAIN

Pain associated with spasticity was reported to respond to BTX-A injections in 21 of 27 patients in the studies cited above:

- shoulder pain in 6 patients;
- wrist pain in 5 patients;
- remainder of patient injection sites were not specified.
- In 187 individuals with pain associated with cervical dystonia, most reported pain relief associated with reduction in dystonia, although the percentage of patients with pain reduction was not specified in every study.
- Not all studies reported positive results: BTX-A was reported to be ineffective in pain attributed to fibromyalgia[4] and pain attributed to chronic pancreatitis.[6] In two cases, a syndrome resembling neuralgic amyotrophy (a painful condition associated with intense sharp or throbbing pain around the shoulder) was reported following BTX-A injections for writer's cramp.[7]

Perhaps the most compelling description of pain relief from BTX-A injections is seen in a report of 30 patients with painful dystonia of Parkinson's disease, "off painful dystonia" (OPD).[5,19] The authors hypothesized that pain of OPD was due to sustained muscle contraction, which causes prolonged muscle spasm. In 30 cases of OPD treated with botulinum toxin, pain improved in all cases within ten days, and in 21 patients' pain completely abated for four months.

26

Remaining Questions

Variables in the cited studies include the presence or absence of concurrent therapy, variable diagnoses, length of time since onset of pain, dosing and concentration, and outcome measurement.

Further studies that control for each of these variables are needed to rigorously measure the putative analgesic effects of BTX-A in the treatment of muscular pain. For example, there is no clear indication in human spasticity research that injection localization of BTX-A is clinically important, yet animal data show superior paralytic effects by injecting BTX-A at motor endplate zones.[20] Future clinical trials might investigate similar responses in myofascial pain by comparing injection locations or toxin concentration.

Conclusions

An existing body of literature in related conditions of muscular hyperactivity provides a rationale for using BTX-A in painful muscular syndromes [1,14,18,21-23], but it is not clear where injections of BTX-A fit into the treatment continuum for myofascial pain. There is evidence to suggest that while BTX-A effectively reduces painful muscular contractions associated with a variety of neurologic disorders, further research is needed to define conditions in which injections might be most effective. The difficulty lies in choosing the appropriate candidate, i.e., finding the patient with painful muscle contractions as the primary source of pain generation. A trial of anesthetic blocking agents might help predict response to subsequent injection of botulinum toxin. Piriformis syndrome may be a good clinical model to study the effects of BTX-A in muscular pain, due to the readily defined clinical features and the isolated location of this structure in relation to other muscles of the low back. Research instruments that incorporate physical measures to quantify the effects of pain, meet criteria similar to self-reported pain scales, and are physiologically relevant should be applied to rigorously examine effects of BTX-A in treatment of painful muscular conditions.[24]

REFERENCES

1. Bhakta BB, Cozens JA, Bamford JM, Chamberlain MA. Use of botulinum toxin in stroke patients with severe upper limb spasticity. J Neurol Neurosurg Psychiatry 1996;61:30-35.
2. Pierson SH, Katz DI, Tarsy D. Botulinum toxin A in the treatment of spasticity: functional implications and patient selection. Arch Phys Med Rehabil 1996;77:717-721.
3. Monsivais JJ, Monsivais DB. Botulinum toxin in painful syndromes. Hand Clinics 1996;12:787-789.
4. Paulson GW, Gill W. Botulinum toxin is unsatisfactory therapy for fibromyalgia. Movement Disorders 1996;11:459-459.
5. Pacchetti C, Albani G, Martignoni E, Godi L, Alfonsi E, Nappi G. "Off" painful dystonia in Parkinson's disease treated with botulinum toxin. Movement Disorders 1995;10:333-336.
6. Sherman S, Kopecky KK, Brashear A, Lehman GA. Percutaneous celiac plexus block with botulinum toxin A did not help the pain of chronic pancreatitis. Journal of Clinical Gastroenterology 1995;20:343-344.
7. Sheean GL, Murray NM, Marsden CD. Pain and remote weakness in limbs injected with botulinum toxin A for writer's cramp. Lancet 1995;346:154-156.
8. Odergren T, Tollback A, Borg J. Efficacy of botulinum toxin for cervical dystonia. A comparison of methods for evaluation. Scand J Rehabil Med 1994;26:191-195.
9. Greene P, Kang U, Fahn S, Brin M, Moskowitz C, Flaster E. Double-blind, placebo-controlled trial of botulinum toxin injections for the treatment of spasmodic torticollis. Neurology 1990;40:1213-1218.
10. Jedynak CP, de Saint Victor JF. [Treatment of spasmodic torticollis by local injections of botulinum toxin]. [French]. Rev Neurol (Paris) 1990;146:440-443.
11. Gelb DJ, Lowenstein DH, Aminoff MJ. Controlled trial of botulinum toxin injections in the treatment of spasmodic torticollis [see comments]. Neurology 1989;39:80-84.
12. Brin MF, Fahn S, Moskowitz C, Friedman A, Shale HM, Greene PE, Blitzer A, List T, Lange D, Lovelace RE, et al. Localized injections of botulinum toxin for the treatment of focal dystonia and hemifacial

spasm. Advances in Neurology 1988;50:599-608.
13. Tsui JK, Fross RD, Calne S, Calne DB. Local treatment of spasmodic torticollis with botulinum toxin. Canadian Journal of Neurological Sciences 1987;14:533-535.
14. Cheshire WP, Abashian SW, Mann JD. Botulinum toxin in the treatment of myofascial pain syndrome [see comments]. Pain 1994;59:65-69.
15. Acquadro MA, Borodic GE. Treatment of myofascial pain with botulinum A toxin [letter]. Anesthesiology 1994;80:705-706.
16. Moore AP, Wood GD. The medical management of masseteric hypertrophy with botulinum toxin type A. British Journal of Oral & Maxillofacial Surgery 1994;32:26-28.
17. Girdler NM. Uses of botulinum toxin [letter; comment]. Lancet 1997;349:953-953.
18. Girdler NM. Use of botulinum toxin to alleviate facial pain [letter]. British Journal of Hospital Medicine 1994;52:363-363.
19. Grazko MA, Polo KB, Jabbari B. Botulinum toxin A for spasticity, muscle spasms, and rigidity. Neurology 1995;45:712-717.
20. Childers MK, Kornegay JN, Aoki R, Otaviani L, Bogan DJ, Petroski G. Evaluating motor end-plate-targeted injections of botulinum toxin type A in a canine model. Muscle Nerve. 1998;21:653-655.
21. Gandhavadi B. Bilateral piriformis syndrome associated with dystonia musculorum deformans. Orthopedics 1990;13:350-351.
22. Johnstone SJ, Adler CH. Headache and facial pain responsive to botulinum toxin: an unusual presentation of blepharospasm. Headache. 1998;38:366-368.
23. Kaufman DM. Use of botulinum toxin injections for spasmodic torticollis of tardive dystonia. Journal of Neuropsychiatry & Clinical Neurosciences 1994;6:50-53.
24. Childers MK, Wilson DJ, Galate JF, Smith BK. Treatment of painful muscle syndromes with botulinum toxin J Back Musc Rehab 10:89-96,1998.

5
CHAPTER

Myofascial Pain Syndromes

The essential features of a myofascial pain syndrome are:

- pain of muscle, soft tissue and fascia,
- static shortening of muscle fibers and associated connective tissue,
- resulting shortening of muscle and connective tissue which may lead to further dysfunction including autonomic disorders and chronic pain,
- lack of confirmatory laboratory or electromyographic studies
- classic myofascial trigger point.[1-5]

THERAPY

A wide variety of therapy is available to patients with myofascial pain syndromes[4-8]. Much of the variation in forms of treatment (and diagnoses) of this disorder probably results from differences in culture, training and recognition of an often undiagnosed syndrome of pain, dysfunction and autonomic dysregulation.

The author, as a specialist in physical medicine and rehabilitation (PM&R), believes that therapeutic exercise is the most powerful tool available to physicians and patients in the treatment of myofascial pain syndromes. Unfortunately, not every patient is able (or willing) to participate in a structured, daily routine of exercise and stretching.

30

When to Consider Botulinum Toxin Type A

For patients with a primary myofascial pain syndrome, the indications for botulinum treatment are not entirely clear.[4;9-11] The author considers patients with primary myofascial pain syndrome as candidates for BTX-A if they have not responded to traditional forms of treatment, have a chronic, refractory problem for three months or longer, have had a complete medical work-up to rule out other non-muscular causes for their pain, and have clearly defined trigger points.

A few words of caution are in order before considering using BTX-A in the treatment of a patient with myofascial pain however. Remember that the approved indications for use of BTX-A in the US are for three conditions: strabismus, blepharospasm and hemifacial spasm.[12] Use of BTX-A for myofascial pain therefore is off-label, and (in the author's opinion) should be considered only for patients with a condition with unsatisfactory results from, or judged inappropriate for, more conservative treatment.

Before considering specific examples however, first turn your consideration to one of the hallmarks of myofascial pain, the trigger point.

TRIGGER POINTS

A myofascial trigger is a local tender point within a taut, ropy band of muscle.[13] While the scientific explanation for exactly what comprises a trigger point is not completely understood, a trigger point has some common characteristic features.

- Pressure (usually with the examiner's fingertip) over a trigger point elicits pain at that area and may also elicit pain at a distance from the point under the fingertip. This is known as "referred pain". Another important feature of the trigger point is that the elicited pain mirrors the patient's experience. Applied pressure often garners the response " Yes, that's the spot!"
- Insertion of a needle, or even a brisk tap with the fingertip, directly over the trigger point may elicit a brisk muscle contraction detectable by the examiner. This brisk contraction of muscle fibers within or around the ropy taut band is termed a "twitch response".[13] In muscles that cross a joint, or large muscles of the hip (like the gluteus maximus), the twitch response is easily seen and may cause the limb to "jump" when the examiner introduces a needle into the trigger point.
- Localized abnormal response from the autonomic nervous system.[14] may cause piloerection, localized sweating or even localized color changes to the skin because of abnormal blood flow.

Typically the muscle containing a trigger point is tight, and difficult or painful for the patient to stretch. This may be most noticeable in certain muscles of the neck, such as the splenius capitus muscle (figure 5-1). In the case of this muscle, the patient may not be able to tilt his head sideways toward the ear as easily as on the opposite side, because of tightness and reduced range-of-movement caused from a taut band.

32

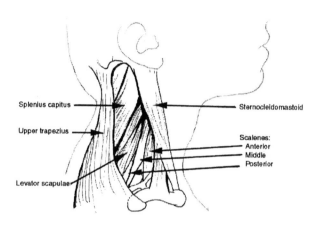

Figure 5-1. Muscles of the neck, lateral aspect.

Spontaneous Electrical Activity

Some researchers think that an abnormal response from the spinal cord causes the trigger point referred pain or twitch response. It also appears that laboratory animals, such as rabbits, may have similar trigger points in some muscles.[13] While rabbits cannot tell scientists where or how much pain is produced when pressure is placed over a trigger point, other evidence makes for a compelling argument about the nature and cause(s) of the trigger point.

Other evidence which supports the idea of the spinal cord (or some portion of the central nervous system) is responsible for the origin of the trigger point comes from electrical studies (electromyography) in humans and laboratory animals. When the tip of a needle electrode is placed very close to an active trigger point, some unusual sounds may be heard from the muscles (much like the heart makes its own characteristic electrical sounds on the EKG). These characteristic sounds are termed "spontaneous electrical activity"[15,16] This spontaneous noise sounds very much like the noise heard from a seashell when placed next to the ear, and is accordingly called the "seashell murmur" by electromyographers.

The importance of this seashell murmur finding in the context of its intimate association with trigger points is that only one structure within muscle is known to create that peculiar sound, and that structure is the motor endplate.[17-19]

While it would seem likely that a muscle spindle would be involved in trigger point physiology as well, since spindles are usually seen in association with motor endplates, there is little evidence to support this idea. One interesting study did report finding a muscle spindle at the site of a trigger point in one patient who had the trigger point site biopsied.[20] However, there seems to be more evidence for a disturbance in the motor endplate itself, rather than a primary spindle problem. Especially since electrical activity (spike potentials) are known to travel a distance along a taut band that exceeds the length of a muscle spindle,[18,21] it seems unlikely that the spindle is ultimately responsible for formation of a trigger point.

Another interesting study examined rabbit muscle after a marker (iron deposit) was placed at precisely the location where an active trigger point was identified by twitch response, taut band, and spontaneous electrical activity. Small "c" nerve fibers (most likely nerves that carry pain information) were found in the immediate vicinity.[13, 20]

Neuromuscular Blocking Agents and Botulinum Toxin Type A Therapy

If abnormal endplate activity does occur, and is indeed responsible for trigger point activity in the myofascial pain syndrome, then a powerful rationale exists for the use of BTX-A in the treatment of myofascial pain syndromes and trigger points.[22] Based upon the idea that pain in this case is due to involuntary muscle contraction, it seems likely that any intervention which (at least temporarily) relieves pain by preventing or reducing muscle contractions might predict how a patient responds to botulinum toxin. However, while trigger point injections or intramuscular compartment blocks by anesthetic agents may predict future response to treatment with botulinum toxin, an eventual problem arises in differentiating the beneficial effects caused from blocking sensory nerves (with anesthetic agents) from the effects produced by BTX-A.

One solution to this problem may be use of atracurium. Atracurium inhibits the excitation-contraction coupling at the myoneural junction by competing with acetylcholine at the nerve terminal.[24] The resulting transient myoneural blockade is deactivated by diffusion from the endplate and degradated into inactive metabolites. Such dual mechanisms of deactivation limit prolonged responses in patients with renal or liver function compromise. The elimination half-life of I.V. atracurium of approximately 22 minutes, with a 95% recovery of myoneural function by 45 minutes. An estimated 82% of I.V. atracurium is plasma protein bound, suggesting that intramuscular injections may preferentially remain local, particularly if given with epinephrine, rather than rapidly diffuse into the bloodstream and other body compartments.

Ed Dunteman, MD, in a personal communication with the author, suggested that since BTX-A's duration of action persists for weeks, there is a need for a specific and sensitive prognostic trial agent which might inhibit muscular contraction for only a short duration, essentially mimicking the effects of botulinum toxin. Short-acting reversible agents would limit undesirable effects of anesthetic agents, such as unwanted weakness, or loss of sensation. Of the available neuromuscular blocking agents, he suggests considering atracurium,[23-25] which has the lowest volume of distribution. Also, since it offers a more limited diffusion injected intramuscularly, injection is preferred to the more commonly used intravenous administration.

Trigger Points Injections with Botulinum Toxin in the Literature

Cheshire et al described responses in six patients with chronic myofascial pain to trigger point injections with

BTX-A in a randomized, double-blind, placebo-controlled study.[10]

- Cervical paraspinal or shoulder girdle trigger points were injected with either saline or 50 units of BTX-A reconstituted in 4 ml saline injected equally in 2 or 3 sites. Responses were measured over 8 weeks by verbal pain descriptors, visual analogue scales, pressure algometer and palpable muscle spasm or firmness.

- Four of six subjects experienced reduction in pain and spasm following botulinum toxin, but not saline, injections. One subject experienced no change by any variables following either treatment, and another subject responded favorably in all variables after both placebo and BTX-A injections.

- Onset of responses occurred within the first week following BTX-A injections, with a mean duration of five-six weeks. The authors concluded that beneficial effects of BTX-A in myofascial pain occurred through the interruption of muscle contraction, and that a larger study was needed to confirm these preliminary findings before treatment could be unequivocally recommended.

In comparison, Wheeler et al conducted a randomized, double-blinded, controlled study comparing injections of normal saline versus injections of 50 and 100 units of BTX-A at trigger points in 23 patients with patients with myofascial pain syndrome. [26]

- The authors found no significant difference in visual analogue pain or disability scores, patients' global assessment of symptoms or in pressure algometer readings throughout four months of follow-up.

- There was a statistical trend towards significant improvement in scores among a small cohort, 39% of the original participants, who were originally treated with BTX-A and then chose to receive a second 100 unit injection.

- Authors speculate there may be a dose-related effect of BTX-A that was not evident in this study and therefore further study may be warranted.

- It is worth mentioning however, that the group receiving second injections contained significantly fewer patients with work-related injuries than the control group.

Identifying Myofascial Pain Syndromes for Botulinum Toxin Type A Therapy

Factors which might identify a pain syndrome as potentially responding favorably to BTX-A injections would include muscle hypertrophy, neurogenic and/or vascular compression, anatomic localization which isolates the target muscle from other structures, and more than one outcome measure to determine efficacy of treatment. Under these criteria, the following three pain syndromes typically qualify:

1. Piriformis muscle syndrome
2. Pronator teres syndrome
3. Thoracic outlet syndrome

PIRIFORMIS MUSCLE SYNDROME

Piriformis muscle syndrome[27-29] is a myofascial pain condition that presents with seemingly bizarre symptoms. Patients are typically female with a recent history of trauma to the buttocks or pelvis (usually from a fall) and complain of a deep seated pain in the buttocks and hip, with radiation into the thigh or even into the leg and foot. These characteristic signs and symptoms are thought to be due to sciatic nerve compression by a contracted, hypertrophic piriformis muscle as the nerve passes through the pelvis. Although some clinicians feel that this diagnosis is controversial, more than 50 peer-reviewed articles clearly define clinical, anatomical and electrophysiological evidence for this distinct condition causing low back and leg pain.[27-34]

On clinical examination, pressure over the buttocks at a point midway between the sacrum and greater trochanter of the hip will reproduce the patients pain complaint. Since the piriformis muscle is so deep, palpation of this trigger point can only be properly performed by rectal or vaginal examination. On the posterior-lateral portion of the rectal (or vaginal) vault, you will find that palpation of the trigger point elicits pain at the site of compression and refers pain either into the thigh or down the leg.

Beatty's manuever[35] is a helpful clinical maneuver to elicit pain in this condition as well. It requires the patient lie on the non-painful side, and abduct the thigh by moving the painful leg off the table.

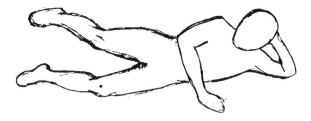

Figure 5-2. Beatty's maneuver.

This maneuver effectively contracts the piriformis muscle and should reproduce patient's pain in the buttocks.

However, since the syndrome essentially causes sciatic nerve compression at the level of the hip, other causes of sciatica should be ruled out (such as a herniated lumbar disc). One helpful diagnostic aid is electromyography. In the case of sciatic neuropathy at the level of the nerve root in the back, the EMG exam should reveal abnormal spontaneous electrical activity in the extensor muscles of the back, while in piriformis syndrome no such abnormal electrical activity should be seen in the back muscles.[36,37] A special nerve conduction test, called the H reflex, may be abnormal in piriformis syndrome when the sciatic nerve is compressed by abduction, internal rotation and flexion of the thigh.

Diagnosis of piriformis syndrome requires:

1. The clinician rule out causes of sciatic neuropathy from compression at the level of the spine (such as a herniated disc, or space-occupying lesion)
2. Pain in the buttocks on compression at a spot

overlying the piriformis muscle, and referral of
pain down the leg
3. Positive Beatty's maneuver.

When to consider Botulinum Toxin Type A

In some cases, conservative treatment of piriformis
syndrome fails, and local injections of anesthetics and/or
steroids may be considered. Surgical resection of the
piriformis muscle is an additional option. However, some
patients may gain short-term benefits from local trigger
point injections into the muscle but remain refractory to
other treatment for long-term pain control. This subset of
patients might benefit from botulinum toxin type A.

To examine the effectiveness of intramuscular BTX-A
injections as a treatment for piriformis muscle syndrome,
the author examined a convenience sample of three
consecutive patients.[38] All patients presented with
findings consistent with a diagnosis of piriformis
syndrome and all failed a trial of conservative
management including non-steroidal anti-inflammatory
agents (NSAIDS), stretching, ultrasound and piriformis
trigger point injections. H-reflexes and segmental nerve
conduction studies in all patients confirmed conduction
block along the sciatic nerve above the gluteal fold,
consistent with the diagnosis.

The involved piriformis muscle in each patient was
injected under fluoroscopic guidance with 100 units of
BTX-A reconstituted in 5ccs of preservative-free saline.
Pain reduction was assessed through pretreatment to
posttreatment differences on a visual analogue scale of
pain intensity, psychologic distress from pain, spasm
frequency, and interference with daily activities. Results

41

of this open label case series demonstrated that the average pain scores decreased from 6.1 to 3.4 and 3.6 two weeks later. Twelve weeks later, two out of three patients had returned to their previous pain levels, whereas one patient sustained longer lasting benefit.

The author is currently conducting a double-blind, placebo controlled crossover study of the effectiveness of BTX-A injection for refractory piriformis syndrome. As of yet, there are no definitive answers for dose, injection location or dilution, but ancedotal evidence and this small case series suggest injections of BTX-A may be beneficial in some chronic, refractory cases.

PRONATOR TERES SYNDROME

Pronator teres syndrome [39-41] is a myofascial pain syndrome variant which is caused from hypertrophy (enlargement) and swelling of the pronator teres muscle resulting in compression of the median nerve near the elbow.

Symptoms depend on the site of compression of the median nerve, thus two types of symptoms may occur. Compression of the median nerve at or just above the elbow leads to weakness of the pronator teres muscle, causing difficulty in rotating the wrist from the "palms up" position to a "palms down" position. Another site of median nerve compression may be at the pronator muscle itself.[42] However, median nerve compression at the pronator teres muscle does not involve the muscle since its innervation comes from another site of the median nerve sparing the pronator teres muscle.

If compression of the median nerve continues long

enough, nerve loss will involve both loss of sensation and weakness of the flexor (palm) side of the forearm. Sensory losses may include the thumb, index and middle fingers, and half the ring finger. Weakness usually involves flexion (inability to make a tight fist) and opposition of the thumb and fingers.

Pain in the distribution of the median nerve is the most significant feature.[40,42] Symptoms are relieved by rest and aggravated by activities such as twisting a screwdriver or opening a jar. Symptoms are reproduced by resisted pronation of the arm.

Nerve conduction studies and electromyography can confirm the diagnosis of pronator teres syndrome by localizing the site of median nerve entrapment.

Treatment Options

Traditional treatment options include:
- Rest
- Modification of activities
- Physical modalities
- Myofascial massage or soft tissue manipulation
- Surgical release of the median nerve

However, since pronator teres syndrome is thought to occur due to muscle hypertrophy, swelling and subsequent nerve compression, it seems a likely candidate for BTX-A therapy. Under the right conditions, local injection of BTX-A into the pronator teres muscle might result in muscle atrophy and subsequent decompression of the median nerve.

THORACIC OUTLET SYNDROME

Thoracic outlet syndrome[4;43] is a myofascial pain syndrome involving compression of the nerves of the brachial plexus and/or the vessels (subclavian artery and vein) of the upper limb. Compression occurs between the neck and the shoulder.

Since the thoracic outlet is bounded by the anterior and middle scalene muscles, the first rib, the clavicle, and (inferiorly) by the tendon of the pectoralis minor muscle, hypertrophy (enlargement) of the scalene muscles may contribute to signs and symptoms of this syndrome.

SCALENE MUSCLES

Scalene anterior muscle:
1. Elevates the first rib in breathing
2. Bends the neck forward and laterally
3. Rotates the neck to the opposite side

Scalene medius muscle:
1. Same as scalene anterior

Scalene posterior muscle:
2. Raises the second rib in breathing
3. Bends the neck laterally
4. May slightly rotate the neck

Signs and Symptoms[44]

Signs and symptoms of thoracic outlet syndrome include:
- Painful sensations in the shoulder and ulnar nerve distribution of the hand
- Adson's test: patient turns head to the involved side,
    - Holds deep breath
    - Raises the chin
    - Clinician palpates the radial pulse
    - Positive test = pulse diminishes & pain reproduced

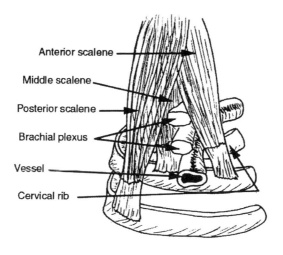

Anterior scalene

Middle scalene

Posterior scalene

Brachial plexus

Vessel

Cervical rib

Figure 5-3. Anatomy of the thoracic outlet

- Roos' test:
  - Patient abducts shoulders 90 degrees, flexes elbows 90 degrees
  - Patient opens/closes hands slowly for three minutes
  - Clinician observes for: hand pallor, diminished pulses, ulnar dysesthesias (all positive for thoracic outlet syndrome)

Other causes of compression (besides muscle hypertrophy) in the thoracic outlet should be considered since the thoracic outlet is an enclosed, relatively small space.

46

Anything that might narrow the space or cause swelling and edema of any of the associated structures:

Other causes of thoracic outlet syndrome include:[44-47]

- Fractured clavicle
- Cervical rib
- Tumor within the thoracic outlet
- Movements which compress the thoracic outlet (shoulder hyperabduction)
- Chest breathing (vs. diaphragm breathing)

Treatment Options [40,48]

Traditional treatment options include:
- Surgical removal of first rib
- Surgical removal of one of the scalene muscles
- Weight loss, postural re-education, shoulder muscle exercises
- Physical modalities for pain relief (heat, cold, e-stim, ultrasound)
- Spinal manipulation

Similar to piriformis and pronator teres syndromes, it is reasonable to consider BTX-A treatment for thoracic outlet syndrome due to scalene muscle hypertrophy. However, special precautions should be considered when injecting the scalene muscles due to the possibility of weakening accessory muscle(s) of respiration, the potential for pneumothorax, and close proximity to vascular/nerve structures. For these reasons, special imaging techniques (CT, fluoro, ultrasound) most likely are warranted.

Injection techniques are described in detail in Chapter 7.

REFERENCES

1. Bennett R. Fibromyalgia, chronic fatigue syndrome, and myofascial pain. [Review] [81 refs]. *Current Opinion in Rheumatology.* 1998;10:95-103.
2. Bohr TW. Fibromyalgia syndrome and myofascial pain syndrome. Do they exist?. [Review] [97 refs]. *Neurologic Clinics.* 1995;13:365-384.
3. Borg-Stein J, Stein J. Trigger points and tender points: one and the same? Does injection treatment help?. [Review] [62 refs]. *Rheumatic Diseases Clinics of North America.* 1996;22:305-322.
4. Fricton JR. Myofascial pain syndrome. [Review] [46 refs]. *Neurologic Clinics.* 1989;7:413-427.
5. McClaflin RR. Myofascial pain syndrome. Primary care strategies for early intervention. [Review] [18 refs]. *Postgraduate Medicine.* 1994;96:56-59.
6. King JC, Goddard MJ. Pain rehabilitation. 2. Chronic pain syndrome and myofascial pain. *Archives.of.Physical.Medicine & Rehabilitation.* 1994;75:Spec-14
7. Snyder-Mackler L, Bork C, Bourbon B, Trumbore D. Effect of helium-neon laser on musculoskeletal trigger points. *Physical Therapy.* 1986;66:1087-1090.
8. Thorsen H, Gam AN, Svensson BH, et al. Low level laser therapy for myofascial pain in the neck and shoulder girdle. A double-blind, cross-over study. *Scandinavian Journal of Rheumatology.* 1992;21:139-141.
9. Acquadro MA, Borodic GE. Treatment of myofascial pain with botulinum A toxin [letter]. *Anesthesiology.* 1994;80:705-706.
10. Cheshire WP, Abashian SW, Mann JD. Botulinum toxin in the treatment of myofascial pain syndrome [see comments]. *Pain.* 1994;59:65-69.
11. Vernick SH. Comments on Cheshire et al. (PAIN, 59 (1994) 65-69) [letter; comment]. *Pain.* 1995;62:249-249.
12. Jankovic J, Brin MF. Therapeutic uses of botulinum toxin. [Review]. NEJM 1991;324:1186-1194.
13. Hong CZ, Simons DG. Pathophysiologic and electrophysiologic mechanisms of myofascial trigger points. [Review] [108 refs]. Archives.of.Physical.Medicine & Rehabilitation. 1998;79:863-872.
14. Fischer AA. Documentation of myofascial trigger points. [Review] [21 refs]. Archives.of.Physical.Medicine & Rehabilitation. 1988;69:286-291.
15. Buchthal F. Spontaneous electrical activity: an overview. [Review]. Muscle Nerve 1982;5:S52-S59
16. Graven-Nielsen T, McArdle A, Phoenix J, Arendt-Nielsen L, Jensen TS, Jackson MJ, Edwards RH. In vivo model of muscle pain:

quantification of intramuscular chemical, electrical, and pressure changes associated with saline- induced muscle pain in humans. Pain 1997;69:137-143.

17. Awad EA. Muscle fiber and motor endplate [letter]. Arch Phys Med Rehabil 1980;61:149-149.

18. Brown WF, Varkey GP. The origin of spontaneous electrical activity at the end-plate zone. Ann Neurol 1981;10:557-560.

19. Childers MK, Kornegay JN, Aoki R, Otaviani L, Bogan DJ, Petroski G. Evaluating motor end-plate-targeted injections of botulinum toxin type A in a canine model. Muscle Nerve 1998;21:653-655.

20. Cazzato G, Walton JN. The pathology of the muscle spindle. A study of biopsy material in various muscular and neuromuscular diseases. Journal of the Neurological Sciences 1968;7:15-70.

21. Pickett JB, Schmidley JW. Sputtering positive potentials in the EMG: an artifact resembling positive waves. Neurology 1980;30:215-218.

22. Childers MK, Wilson DJ, Galate JF, Smith BK. Treatment of painful muscle syndromes with botulinum toxin. j back musculoskel rehabil 1997;in press:

23. Owens CA, Brakoniecki J. - Cisatracurium: a new nondepolarizing neuromuscular blocking agent. [Review] [22 refs]. - Connecticut Medicine 1996 Aug;60(8):461-3 461-33.

24. May JR, Rutkowski AF. - The role of nondepolarizing neuromuscular blocking agents in mechanically ventilated patients. [Review] [16 refs]. - Journal of the Medical Association of Georgia 1994 Aug;83(8):473-6, 484 1899;473-476.

25. Torda TA. - The 'new' relaxants. A review of the clinical pharmacology of atracurium and vecuronium. [Review] [108 refs]. - Anaesthesia & Intensive Care 1987 Feb;15(1):72-82 72-822.

26. Wheeler AH, Goolkasian P, Gretz SS. A randomized, double-blind, prospective pilot study of botulinum toxin injection for refractory, unilateral, cervicothoracic, paraspinal, myofascial pain syndrome. Spine 1998 Aug ; 23(15):1662-1666

27. Solheim LF, Siewers P, Paus B. The piriformis muscle syndrome. Sciatic nerve entrapment treated with section of the piriformis muscle. *Acta Orthopaedica Scandinavica*. 1981;52:73-75.

28. Simons DG, Travell JG. Myofascial origins of low back pain. 3. Pelvic and lower extremity muscles. *Postgraduate Medicine*. 1983;73:99-105, 108.

29. Hallin RP. Sciatic pain and the piriformis muscle. *Postgraduate Medicine*. 1983;74:69-72.

30. Steiner C, Staubs C, Ganon M, Buhlinger C. Piriformis syndrome: pathogenesis, diagnosis, and treatment. *Journal of the American Osteopathic Association*. 1987;87:318-323.

31. Noftal F. The Piriformis Syndrome. *Canadian Journal of Surgery*. 1988;31:210-210.

32. Julsrud ME. Piriformis syndrome. *Journal of the American Podiatric Medical Association*. 1989;79:128-131.

33. Jankiewicz JJ, Hennrikus WL, Houkom JA. The appearance of the piriformis muscle syndrome in computed tomography and magnetic

resonance imaging. A case report and review of the literature. [Review] [24 refs]. *Clin Orthop Rel Res.* 1991;205-209.

34. Fishman LM, Zybert PA. Electrophysiologic evidence of piriformis syndrome. *Arch Phys Med Rehabil.* 1992;73:359-364.

35. Beatty RA. The piriformis muscle syndrome: a simple diagnostic maneuver [see comments]. *Neurosurg.* 1994;34:512-4; discuss.

36. LaBan MM, Meerschaert JR, Taylor RS. Electromyographic evidence of inferior gluteal nerve compromise: an early representation of recurrent colorectal carcinoma. *Arch Phys Med Rehabil.* 1982;63:33-35.

37. Papadopoulos SM, McGillicuddy JE, Albers JW. Unusual cause of 'piriformis muscle syndrome'. *Archives of Neurology.* 1990;47:1144-1146.

38. Galate JF, Childers MK, Gnatz S. Effectiveness of botulinum toxin in refractory piriformis muscle syndrome. *Arch Phys Med Rehabil.* 1997;78:1041(Abstract)

39. Gainor BJ. Modified exposure for pronator syndrome decompression: a preliminary experience. *Orthopedics.* 1993;16:1329-1331.

40. Olehnik WK, Manske PR, Szerzinski J. Median nerve compression in the proximal forearm. *Journal of Hand Surgery - American Volume.* 1994;19:121-126.

41. Tsai TM, Syed SA. A transverse skin incision approach for decompression of pronator teres syndrome. *Journal of Hand Surgery - British Volume.* 1994;19:40-42.

42. Tulwa N, Limb D, Brown RF. Median nerve compression within the humeral head of pronator teres. *Journal of Hand Surgery - British Volume.* 1994;19:709-710.

43. Sucher BM. Thoracic outlet syndrome--a myofascial variant: Part 2. Treatment. [Review] [17 refs]. *Journal of the American Osteopathic Association.* 1990;90:810-812.

44. Pang D, Wessel HB. Thoracic outlet syndrome. [Review] [159 refs]. *Neurosurg.* 1988;22:105-121.

45. Bland JH. Cervical and thoracic pain including thoracic outlet syndrome and brachial neuritis. [Review] [24 refs]. *Current Opinion in Rheumatology.* 1990;2:242-252.

46. Brown HS, Smith RA. First rib resection for neurovascular syndromes of the thoracic outlet. [Review] [39 refs]. *Surgical Clinics of North America.* 1974;54:1277-1289.

47. Dobrusin R. An osteopathic approach to conservative management of thoracic outlet syndromes. [Review] [20 refs]. *Journal of the American Osteopathic Association.* 1989;89:1046-1050.

48. Barton PM. Piriformis syndrome: a rational approach to management. *Pain.* 1991;47:345-352.

6

CHAPTER

Muscle Spindles and Disordered Motor Control

Muscle spindles are special sensory structures called mechanoreceptors that respond to physical changes in muscle length. Muscle spindles are made of small spindle-shaped muscle fibers called intrafusal muscle fibers because they are found within ordinary, extrafusal skeletal muscle fibers. The spindles are clustered in small bundles surrounded by a protective fluid-filled capsule and lie in parallel with extrafusal fibers. Figure 6-1 shows a microscopic photo of a muscle spindle.

Muscle spindles may be thought of as space-saving devices. Using information from the spindle, the spinal cord can help regulate muscle tension and position without having to transmit information all the way to the brain. The ends of the muscle spindles are connected to tendon, connective tissue or extrafusal muscle fibers. When the entire muscle is stretched, tension is placed on the spindle apparatus. Since the muscle spindle is also connected to sensory nerve endings, called 1a afferents, stretching results in activation of the spindle sensory endings. The sensory component (found in the middle part of the spindle) responds to changes in muscle length.

51

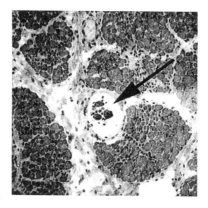

Figure 6-1. Micrograph from skeletal muscle, transverse 10μ cyrosection. Arrow points to a muscle spindle. Note the clear area (fluid filled capsule) which surrounds the spindle. Stain: H&E. Magnification: 20X. Source: author.

Once the spinal cord receives information that the spindles have been stretched, a special motor neuron, the gamma motor neuron (relaying signals from the spinal cord to the ends of the spindle) causes the muscle spindle to contract, and subsequently "resets" the sensory nerve. In a way, the gamma motor neuron acts like a thermostat to control how sensitive the sensory structure is to changes in the length of the muscle.

Muscle Spindle's Relation to Painful Muscle Conditions

There appears to be little evidence that painful muscle areas, such as trigger points, are associated with a structural change or sensory structure such as the muscle spindle. However, in certain conditions of abnormal muscle activity, the spindle is intimately involved. In the spastic condition, for example, the stretch reflex is enhanced due to a variety of reasons, such as a lack of inhibition from spinal cord interneurons. Whatever the reason, muscle spindle physiology in the spastic condition is an important regulator of muscle tone.

Pain is often associated with spasticity, and this topic is explored in detail below. While not clearly understood, or rigorously tested, an association can be made between abnormal spindle physiology and painful muscular conditions or "muscle spasms". It has been the author's clinical observation that BTX-A at doses lower than anticipated for relief of hypertonia are effective for the relief of pain associated with spasticity or dystonia. One could speculate that these lower doses may be enough to effectively weaken or "reset" the intrinsic (spindle) fibers, and thus, indirectly result in pain relief.

Therefore, the idea behind the use of BTX-A for some painful conditions is that pain relief may result from not only local muscle paralysis but by a decrease in the reflex muscle tone.

Implications of Botulinum Toxin Type A as a Modifier of Spindle Discharge

While there is yet to be definitive evidence based on humans, if BTX-A does modify spindle discharge, then painful muscle syndromes that are regulated by spindle physiology might be effectively treated through local injections. Experiments in rats [1,2] have shown that BTX-A reduces spindle discharge, probably by altering the sensitivity of spindle physiology. As a result of such altered physiology, BTX-A may cause changes in the way muscles are activated by either volitional control, or by altering an abnormal central programming.

Also, there is evidence to suggest treatments that increase spindle activity may enhance uptake of BTX-A into muscles. In an experiment by Hesse et al, [3] ten patients with lower limb spasticity were treated with BTX-A injections and evaluated by computer gait analysis and clinical measures of muscle tone. The difference between the two groups was that one group received electrical stimulation to muscles of the lower leg six times each day for three days after BTX-A injection while the other group received only injections. Results showed superior improvement in the group of patients receiving electrical stimulation compared to the group receiving injections alone.

Electrical stimulation causes muscles to contract, and effectively stretches muscle fibers. One example of the use of electrical stimulation can be seen in patients with spinal paralysis. Patients with complete paralysis from spinal cord injury can actually maintain their muscle mass by using electrical stimulation regularly. Another example can be seen in the use of electrical stimulation in rehabilitation of athletes following knee surgery. Electrical stimulation might similarly be effective when used in combination with BTX-A for painful muscle syndromes.

Since muscle spindles are protected by a thick, fluid-filled capsule, uptake of BTX-A in spindles likely occurs by a specific acceptor.[4] Rosales et al [1] demonstrated increased vulnerability to the effects of BTX-A in spindle endings which contained bag 1 fibers (spindles contain nerve endings of three types, termed bag 1, bag 2, and chain). The important point here, is that bag 1 endings are most active during dynamic (active) stretching. Theoretically, treatments (like electrical stimulation, or active stretching activities) might enhance the clinical effects of BTX-A injections in painful syndromes.

Static Stretching

The author has occasionally prescribed a modality known as "inhibitory casting" following BTX-A treatment for severe spasticity. The idea being that cast application provides low-load, long duration stretch on spastic muscles,[6-8] and thus alters the activity of the spindle for a finite time. One way in which spindle activity is supposedly measured, is by performing an electrophysiologic test known as "vibratory inhibition of the H reflex". The author's research[5] measuring H reflex inhibition during casting lends support to the idea that during application of an inhibitory cast, motor neuron excitability (probably mediated by the spindle) is decreased in the spastic upper limb.

Other related research[9] also supports this theory by demonstrating alpha motor neuron reflex inhibition following application of circumferential pressure in subjects with spinal cord injury. Thus, some treatments that involve static stretching (versus dynamic or active stretching), when performed during the first few hours of administration of BTX-A might paradoxically inhibit the desirable paralytic effects of the toxin. Although these studies tend to support the use of static stretching in the spastic condition, timing with BTX-A administration may be important. While more research is needed to establish the usefulness and timing of casting (or static stretching) in combination with the treatment of spasticity and painful muscle conditions, this modality might be useful as an adjunctive therapy when prescribed a few days after initial injection.

SPASTICITY

Spasticity is a term given to describe a condition associated with abnormal muscle tone due to an abnormality of the central nervous system. Specifically, spasticity [10] is considered to be a hallmark of an upper motor neuron syndrome (as opposed to a lower motor neuron syndrome).

The upper motor neuron syndrome consists of features such as
- spasticity
- clonus
- increased reflexes
- dystonia
- weakness
- lack of dexterity
- slowness in the initiation of movement

If a patient presents with abnormal muscle tone and findings which are not consistent with an upper motor neuron syndrome, spasticity would not be considered the appropriate term to describe the condition. In fact, while some physiology literature uses the terms spasticity and dystonia interchangeably, from a clinical standpoint dystonia[11] refers to a type of disorder of movement that usually is not seen within the context of an upper motor neuron syndrome. As would be expected, treatment of dystonia is quite different from the treatment of spasticity.

Spasticity may be manifested in the patient as abnormal resistance to movement. For example, when the patient's gamma motor neuron is overly sensitive to stretch tension ("gamma" spasticity), on examination the faster you attempt to move the spastic limb, the more resistance you encounter. This is termed "velocity-dependent" muscle resistance. In addition to observing velocity-dependent muscle resistance, you should see signs of the upper motor neuron syndrome (brisk reflexes, weakness and lack of dexterity). Spasticity is not seen in patients with normal central nervous system physiology, and should not be confused with "muscle spasm".

Muscle spasm is not a specifically defined medical term, and generally refers to pain associated with muscle injury or in the context of a myofascial pain syndrome. Most people are familiar with a back muscle "spasm" or muscle "cramp". These involuntary contractions of individual muscles or groups of muscles may come on suddenly, without warning, and be excruciatingly painful. Muscle spasm may be related to irritability of the muscle spindle or due to a temporary electrolyte imbalance (such as seen after vigorous athletic training). The important point is that while muscle spasms are not related to spasticity per se, muscle spasms may occur in patients with spasticity. Pain associated with spasticity may be related to muscle spasm, and not necessarily related to the increased muscle tone due to a problem in the central nervous system.

Antispastic Agents and Pain Relief

This is a complex topic. Simply stated, agents which either decrease motor neuron excitability[3,12-15] or increase the inhibitory influence on the alpha motor neuron,[16,17] reduce muscle tone and thereby may reduce pain associated with muscular hyperactivity.

Some antispastic agents work by increasing the inhibitory influence of the amino acid called GABA,[18] which in turn either: activates chloride channels (hyperpolarizes the postsynaptic membrane making it "harder" to depolarize) or activates cAMP which decreases intracellular calcium ions required for muscle contraction.

The antispastic agent, <u>dantrolene sodium</u>,[19] acts directly on the muscle contractile mechanism by decreasing the availability of intracellular calcium.

Other agents, <u>tizanadine</u>, and <u>clonidine</u> (alpha 2 adrenergic agonists) presumably act by mechanisms which increase noradrenergic inhibition to reduce motor neuron excitability.[18,20]

Botulinum Toxin Type A as Therapy for Spasticity

BTX-A may work in (gamma) spasticity by peripheral mechanisms rather than by central mechanisms of increasing inhibition.[21-23] In patients with hemiplegic spasticity, for example, BTX-A injections into spastic calf muscles presumably act by focally weakening extrafusal muscle fibers. The functional result in improved walking ability occurs by allowing the spastic leg to roll over the ankle with less resistance to abnormal spastic contractions.

There is indirect evidence[1] to suggest that BTX-A might also have an even greater paralytic effect on the intrafusal fibers of muscle spindle compared to extrafusal fibers in spastic patients. This property of greater paralytic effect on the spindle fibers may be useful to the clinician in the treatment of spasticity. If weakening the muscle spindle fibers in the patient with spasticity would decrease the spindle afferent discharge, then a reduced hyperactive stretch reflex should be observed in spastic patients. This putative property of BTX-A is particularly desirable in the setting of a patient with hemiplegic gait with ankle clonus.

Clinical Evidence In Spasticity Literature

There is evidence that the paralytic properties of BTX-A are enhanced in patients given electrical stimulation to spastic muscles during the first few days after injection with botulinum toxin.[14,21,24] Some experts speculate that the enhanced activity of BTX-A is due to increased spindle discharge from electrical stimulation.

BTX-A might also be useful to the clinician in the treatment of patients with spasticity accompanied by painful spasms. For while oral antispastic agents also may be helpful in reducing the pain related to spasticity and muscle spasms, many patients cannot tolerate side effects of these agents (sedation, weakness, etc.). It is the author's experience that doses of botulinum toxin, (at doses even lower than required to reduce spasticity), injected into painful muscles have analgesic effects. This experience is also seen in reports of pain reduction from BTX-A use in spasticity literature.

Also, the author believes that information gained from spasticity cases might be applicable to patients with myofascial pain, as similar mechanisms may contribute to painful spasms whether due to spasticity or other reasons. While controversial, the trigger point (seen in myofascial pain syndromes) may be associated with abnormal spindle function.[25,26] In this scenario, overactive spindle mechanisms might respond effectively to local injections of BTX-A resulting in decreased outflow to extrafusal fibers and subsequent diminished spasm.

DYSTONIA

Dystonia is a condition which causes involuntary muscular contraction, often resulting in bizarre twisting postures.[11] It was first termed, "dystonia musculorum deformans" by Oppenheim to describe the progressive nature of the twisting movements that often led to deforming postures.

The most common cause of dystonia is idiopathic, with or without a hereditary pattern. Other causes include head trauma, peripheral injury, stroke and encephalitis.[27]

Focal dystonias affect only one segment or area of the body. Most of us are familiar with focal dystonia of the neck muscles which cause rotation (torticollis).[28] Other forms of focal dystonia include involuntary eye closing (blepharospasm), writer's cramp, and spastic speech (spasmotic dysphonia).

Dystonia and Pain

Some investigators have reported that as many as 70% of patients with some forms of cervical dystonia [29] have pain associated with involuntary muscle contraction. Other forms of focal dystonias are also associated with pain that is thought to arise from involuntary contraction of muscles.[30-32]

Diagnosis

Typically, neurologists with special training and interests in movement disorders treat the dystonias. Since most dystonias are diagnosed by clinical evaluation, it is important that any patient considered to have an undiagnosed dystonia be evaluated by a specialist with experience and training in movement disorders.

To find a movement disorder specialist in your area, contact:

Dystonia Medical Research Foundation.
One East Wacker Drive, Suite 2430
Chicago,IL 60601-1905 USA
-800-377-3978, or 312-755-0198.
www.dystonia-foundation.org/

Treatment

There is no single agent (systemic or local) that is uniformly effective in the treatment of all dystonias. Many movement disorder experts feel that the treatment of choice for focal dystonias are local injections of botulinum toxin.[30,33-36]

Before determining treatment however, one must confirm a diagnosis of focal dystonia as opposed to a myofascial pain syndrome. One clue may be that most dystonias result in twisting postures, are worse with voluntary movement or stress, and are insidious in onset. However, the author has seen a few patients with involuntary muscular contractions of the trapezius, levator scapulae and various shoulder girdle muscles that did not result in the stereotypical dystonic limb postures. However, the patients did present with pain, muscle hypertrophy, frustration with prior (ineffective) medical treatment for the relief of pain, and involuntary muscle contractions found on EMG exam.

Electromyography (EMG) may be helpful in sorting out pain arising from muscular "spasm" and pain arising from the involuntary muscular contractions associated with dystonia. Pain associated with the latter may be managed most effectively with local injections of botulinum toxin, whereas the former may be amenable to other treatment. Consider a consultation with a neurologist or physiatrist for EMG in these cases.

Other research has shown that abnormal muscle contractions seen in dystonia can be modified by blocking afferent nerves, (signals going from the spinal cord toward the muscle), with local injections of lidocaine. Patients with dystonia often learn to take advantage of "sensory tricks" which similarly alter abnormal muscle activity.

In summary, the idea behind the use of BTX-A for some painful conditions is that pain relief may result from not only local muscle paralysis but by a decrease in the reflex muscle tone.

REFERENCES

1.   Rosales RL, Arimura K, Takenaga S, Osame M. Extrafusal and intrafusal muscle effects in experimental botulinum toxin-A injection. Muscle Nerve 1996;19:488-496.
2.   Filippi GM, Errico P, Santarelli R, Bagolini B, Manni E. Botulinum A toxin effects on rat jaw muscle spindles. Acta Oto-Laryngologica 1993;113:400-404.

3. Hesse S, Jahnke MT, Luecke D, Mauritz KH. Short-term electrical stimulation enhances the effectiveness of Botulinum toxin in the treatment of lower limb spasticity in hemiparetic patients. Neuroscience Letters 1995;201:37-40.
4. Black JD, Dolly JO. Selective location of acceptors for botulinum neurotoxin A in the central and peripheral nervous systems. Neuroscience 1987;23:767-779.
5. Barnard P, Dill H, Eldredge P, Held J, Judd D, Nalette E. Reducation of hypertonicity by early casting in a comatose head-injured individual: A case report. *Physical Therapy*. 1984;64:1540-1542.
6. Hill J. The effects of casting on upper extremity motor disorders after brain injury. *Am J Occup Ther*. 1993;48:219-223.
7. Robichaud JA, Agostinucci J. Air-splint pressure effect on soleus muscle alpha motoneuron reflex excitability in subjects with spinal cord injury. *Arch Phys Med Rehabil*. 1996;77:778-782.
8. Childers MK, Biswas S, Petroski G, Merveille O. Casting modulates vibratory inhibition of the H reflex in the spastic upper limb. Arch Phys Med Rehabil 1998;submitted:
9. Glenn MB, Rosenthal M. Rehabilitation following severe traumatic brain injury. Sem Neurol 1985;5:233
10. Bajd T, Bowman B. Testing and modelling of spasticity. J Biomed Eng 1982;4:90
11. Fahn S. - The varied clinical expressions of dystonia. [Review] [47 refs]. - Neurologic Clinics 1984 Aug;2(3):541-54 541-544.
12. Botte MJ, Abrams RA, Bodine-Fowler SC. Treatment of acquired muscle spasticity using phenol peripheral nerve blocks. [Review] [139 refs]. Orthopedics 1995;18:151-159.
13. Herman R. The myotatic reflex. Clinico-physiological aspects of spasticity and contracture. Brain 1970;93:273-312.
14. Price R, Lehmann JF, Boswell-Bessette S, Burleigh A, deLateur BJ. Influence of cryotherapy on spasticity at the human ankle. Arch Phys Med Rehabil 1993;74:300-304.
15. Priebe MM, Sherwood AM, Thornby JI, Kharas NF, Markowski J. Clinical assessment of spasticity in spinal cord injury: a multidimensional problem. Arch Phys Med Rehabil 1996;77:713-716.
16. Seib TP, Price R, Reyes MR, Lehmann JF. The quantitative measurement of spasticity: effect of cutaneous electrical stimulation. Arch Phys Med Rehabil 1994;75:746-750.
17. Tona JL, Schneck CM. The efficacy of upper extremity inhibitive casting: a single- subject pilot study. Am J Occup Ther 1993;47:901-910.
18. Davidoff RA. Antispasticity drugs: mechanisms of action. [Review]. Ann Neurol 1985;17:107-116.
19. Anderson IL, Jones EW. Porcine malignant hyperthermia: effect of dantrolene sodium on in-vitro halothane-induced contraction of susceptible muscle. Anesthesiology 1976;44:57-61.
20. Young RR, Delwaide PJ. Drug therapy: spasticity (first of two parts). NEJM 1981;304:28-33.
21. Hesse S, Krajnik J, Luecke D, Jahnke MT, Gregoric M, Mauritz KH.

Ankle muscle activity before and after botulinum toxin therapy for lower limb extensor spasticity in chronic hemiparetic patients. Stroke 1996;27:455-460.

22. Lagueny A, Burbaud P. [Mechanism of action, clinical indication and results of treatment of botulinum toxin]. [Review] [37 refs] [French]. Neurophysiologie Clinique 1996;26:216-226.

23. Yablon SA, Agana BT, Ivanhoe CB, Boake C. Botulinum toxin in severe upper extremity spasticity among patients with traumatic brain injury: an open-labeled trial. Neurology 1996;47:939-944.

24. Hesse S, Lucke D, Malezic M, Bertelt C, Friedrich H, Gregoric M, Mauritz KH. Botulinum toxin treatment for lower limb extensor spasticity in chronic hemiparetic patients. J Neurol Neurosurg Psychiatry 1994;57:1321-1324.

25. Hong CZ, Hsueh TC. Difference in pain relief after trigger point injections in myofascial pain patients with and without fibromyalgia [see comments]. Archives.of.Physical.Medicine & Rehabilitation. 1996;77:1161-1166.

26. Hong CZ, Simons DG. Pathophysiologic and electrophysiologic mechanisms of myofascial trigger points. [Review] [108 refs]. Archives.of.Physical.Medicine & Rehabilitation. 1998;79:863-872.

27. Markham CH. - The dystonias. [Review] [56 refs]. - Current Opinion in Neurology & Neurosurgery 1992 Jun;5(3):301-7 301-377.

28. Tsui JK, Fross RD, Calne S, Calne DB. Local treatment of spasmodic torticollis with botulinum toxin. Canadian Journal of Neurological Sciences 1987;14:533-535.

29. Odergren T, Tollback A, Borg J. Efficacy of botulinum toxin for cervical dystonia. A comparison of methods for evaluation. Scand J Rehabil Med 1994;26:191-195.

30. Brin MF, Fahn S, Moskowitz C, Friedman A, Shale HM, Greene PE, Blitzer A, List T, Lange D, Lovelace RE, et al. Localized injections of botulinum toxin for the treatment of focal dystonia and hemifacial spasm. Advances in Neurology 1988;50:599-608.

31. Pacchetti C, Albani G, Martignoni E, Godi L, Alfonsi E, Nappi G. "Off" painful dystonia in Parkinson's disease treated with botulinum toxin. Movement Disorders 1995;10:333-336.

32. Pullman sl, Greene P, Fahn S, Pedersen SF. Approach to the treatment of limb disorders with botulinum toxin A. Experience with 187 patients. Archives of Neurology 1996;53:617-624.

33. Calne S. Local treatment of dystonia and spasticity with injections of botulinum-A toxin. Axone 1993;14:85-88.

34. Grandas F. [Clinical application of botulinum toxin]. [Review] [141 refs] [Spanish]. Neurologia 1995;10:224-233.

35. Hughes AJ. Botulinum toxin in clinical practice. [Review] [15 refs]. Drugs 1994;48:888-893.

36. Jankovic J, Schwartz K, Donovan DT. Botulinum toxin treatment of cranial-cervical dystonia, spasmodic dysphonia, other focal dystonias and hemifacial spasm. J Neurol Neurosurg Psychiatry 1990;53:633-639.

7
CHAPTER

Equipment and Injection Techniques

Therapy with botulinum toxin type A should be individualized for both the patient and the clinician. Equipment needs may be determined by patient needs, clinician's training and the anatomic target for injection. For example, treatments for blepharospasm are usually given by simple subcutaneous injections around the eye, without the use of special equipment. However, injections into the deep compartments of the low back, such as the psoas major muscle compartment, may require the use of special imaging techniques.

The author does not see the need for use of operating rooms or special procedure (sterile) rooms equipped with monitoring devices for the purpose of intramuscular injections of BTX-A using small caliber needles. Most patients can be safely treated in an office setting by experienced clinicians.

For most limb muscles, the author recommends use of electromyography (EMG) or motor point stimulation (e-stim) to identify muscles, particularly the smaller muscles in the forearm. For example, a commonly injected finger flexor muscle, the flexor digitorum sublimis (FDS), is nearly impossible to locate without EMG guidance.[1]

For the clinician who is developing his/her skills in identifying specific muscles for injection with botulinum toxin, the use of simple "audio-only" EMG may further enhance the clinician's understanding of functional anatomy and aid in the decision-making on injection localization.[2-4]

To summarize, here is a list of special equipment to consider for specific parts of the body:

Face:	None required
Neck:	Audio EMG; e-stim
Limbs:	Audio EMG; e-stim
Easily Accessible Trigger Points:	None required
Deep Compartment Muscles of Back:	Fluoroscopy, ultrasound CT and/or EMG
Superficial Muscles Of the Trunk:	Audio EMG
Flexors of Distal Finger Joints:	E-stim

Information on portable audio EMG units and stimulators is found in Appendix A.

As with any procedure in medicine, it will be important for you to get some "hands on" training by an experienced clinician prior to treating patients with BTX-A by injection for the first time. One medical academy has published training guidelines for physicians who use BTX-A to treat neurological disorders. The author strongly encourages attending training seminars and acquiring some one-on-one instruction before proceeding to treat patients with botulinum toxin.

INJECTION LOCATIONS

The electrophysiologic evidence discussed earlier supports an association with abnormal endplate activity and myofascial trigger points. The author's research[5] in dogs and other research in mice[4] support injection techniques that either localize motor endplates or place the injection needle in close proximity to motor endplates. Since trigger points should lie in the close proximity to motor endplates[6,7], the clinician should attempt to target injections toward the zone or distribution of the motor endplates whenever possible. This is the technique the author employs whenever possible. Although it may seem that attempting to localize such small, discrete areas within a large muscle is much like hunting for a needle in a haystack, there are ways in which you can narrow down the likely location of these discrete points.

It has been shown that endplates do not occur randomly scattered throughout skeletal muscle, but occur in groups or "bands" in most cases. The distribution of these locations is relatively well described in humans, and likely coincides with "motor point" maps[8,9] published elsewhere. Motor points are areas within muscle where small motor nerves terminate and are used to direct locations for phenol or alcohol blocks.

Localizing Motor Endplates

As the practicality of localizing motor endplates may be problematic, the equipment mentioned earlier is quite useful. To localize motor endplates, you need to use EMG and additionally have some idea where to start searching within a large muscle. In the case of the trigger point, your

67

task should be somewhat simpler, as you should be able to accurately find the trigger point with the tip of your finger.

Next, connect the EMG to a dual-purpose needle electrode and search for the characteristic noise of the motor endplate. In the case where trigger points are not present, you will need to refer to a motor point chart, or review information on motor endplate zones in Chapter 3 to increase your chances of finding them. Remember, that this technique may not be appropriate in all cases, such as when the patient cannot completely relax the muscle and create electrical silence, or in the case of strap muscles (discussed below) where endplate "zones" don't really apply.

The motor endplate also is home to the neuromuscular junction. Find the motor endplate, and you've localized the neuromuscular junction. For a more detailed description of the characteristic electrophysiologic features of the motor endplate, read Wiederholt's description of the motor endplate.[10-12] In short, the characteristic features of the motor endplate are as follows:

- A low-voltage increase in the baseline of about 10-40 µV (the audio EMG sounds similar to holding a seashell to your ear);
- Usually accompanying irregularly firing monophasic spike discharges.
- Characteristic deep pain described by the patient.

Once one motor endplate has been localized within the target muscle, the author usually does not hunt for others (because of time issues) but rather assumes that he is within the zone or proximity of other motor endplates. Three of four sites are subsequently injected (as illustrated in later sections) in a pattern that likely coincides with the midpoint of the muscle fibers. This technique has been confirmed experimentally in dogs, but not in humans, and there are practical issues that need to be confirmed by future clinical research.

If there is too much noise due to involuntary muscle activity, consider another injection method, such as the motor point method[9,13] or the anatomic method.

Motor point method

You cannot localize motor endplates (the site of action of botulinum toxin) using electromyography unless the patient is able to completely relax the muscle. Some clinicians feel that they can find the motor endplate using electrical stimulation (either with a needle or surface electrode). However, you may not be entirely correct in assuming that motor endplates and motor "points" are one and the same.[14] There is evidence which shows that motor points (localized with a stimulator) in some muscles are actually places in muscle where small motor nerve endings enters into a portion of the muscle, rather than a motor endplate where the chemical (acetylcholine) responsible for muscle contraction is released. However, in other muscles, the motor point overlies the motor endplate. Since the site of action of BTX-A is at the motor endplate, it is important to be able to localize this area within large muscles, but motor points are probably reasonably close, and may be a good alternative in some situations. If you want to explore this technique further, the author suggests reviewing references listed in the bibliography and offers the following summary of earlier research [15]examining the association between motor endplates and motor points in muscle biopsies.

Muscles with long fibers where motor endplates overlies the motor point:

- Biceps
- Deltoid
- Flexor carpi radialis
- Flexor digitorum sublimis
- Vastus internus
- Sternomastoid
- Palmaris longus

The reason for this association between the motor point and motor endplate is due to the parallel arrangement of long muscle fibers (dashed lines) resulting in a linear innervation band ('X'). This band of motor endplates (an "endplate zone") crosses the surface of the muscle at its approximate center:

```
------------------------X------------------------
------------------------X------------------------
------------------------X------------------------
------------------------X------------------------
```

Muscles in which the motor point overlies the motor endplates:

- Tibialis anterior

70

- Brachio-radialis

In these muscles, the muscle fibers arise from superficial connective tissue and run deep towards a muscle-tendon junction, therefore the motor endplates underlie the motor point deep to the surface.

Muscles in which the motor point is proximal to the motor endplates:

- Gastrocnemius
- Peroneus longus

In these muscles, the motor point is proximal to the motor endplate because the muscle fibers receive their innervation several inches distal to the motor point. The motor nerve enters these muscles proximally, and runs along the line of tendon insertion, becoming progressively more superficial. For these reasons, the motor point is easily found at a site superficial and proximal to the motor endplates.

Equipment for motor point localization:

- Peripheral nerve stimulator
- Surface electrodes or single probe stimulator
- Electrode gel
- Dual purpose needle electrode

(Surface) Motor point localization technique:

(Stimulation intensity 5-10 mAmp and 0.5 sec duration.)

71

- Use surface electrode or probe over muscle belly.
- Observe for muscular contraction coincident with stimulation pulse.
- Continue to reduce current until a minimal contraction seen.
- Repeat until the lowest intensity stimulation causes a muscle contraction over one point overlying the muscle, and mark that point on the skin.

Intramuscular motor point localization technique:

- Repeat procedure above intramuscularly:
- Sterilize skin
- Attach lead from needle to cathode (black pole)
- Attach anode (read pole) lead to surface electrode near site of needle entry
- Insert needle through skin at point previously marked
- Turn stimulator on and increase intensity to 3 or 4 mAmp.
- Reduce stim intensity and probe muscle until a contraction can be observed with only 1 mAmp or less.

E-stim and Stretching

Since there is indirect evidence to support the contention that overactive spindle activity enhances the paralytic property of botulinum toxin,[16,17] treatments such as electrical stimulation or muscle stretching, which enhance spindle activity, likely would enhance the effects of the toxin.

***E-stim or stretching after BTX-A injection would
include:***

- Active stretching of injected muscles several
  times each day for 72 hours following injection
  with BTX-A may enhance treatment effects
- Electrical stimulation given several times each
  day for 72 hours following injection may also
  enhance effects
- TENS (transcutaneous electrical neuromuscular
  stimulation) units can easily be programmed to do
  this.

Sample prescription post botulinum toxin

<u>Patient</u>: John Smith
<u>Diagnosis</u>: myofascial pain syndrome, spasticity due
to stroke, etc.

<u>Physical Therapist</u>:
1. "Trial of TENS, post BTX-A injection
Apply electrodes over motor points of injected
muscles and stimulate six times daily (30 minutes) for
three days"
2. "Develop and instruct in a supervised home
stretching program."
3. "Please treat three times per week for two weeks
and provide a report of response to treatment."

TENS Unit

A TENS unit can be used to localize the surface motor
point over a muscle quite easily: attach one surface

electrode onto the patient's skin, and the other electrode on the back of your own hand. Use a little electrode gel or water and gently run your index finger over the surface of the skin overlying the muscle of interest. Adjust the intensity of the TENS unit until you can actually feel the current beneath your finger, then, decrease the stimulus intensity until you no longer can feel any current except for one point on the skin. This point will correspond to the motor point found using the more traditional technique. If you like, you can verify this by increasing the TENS intensity high enough to elicit a muscle contraction over the tip of your finger!

EMG activity method

EMG activity method is yet another method to target injections of BTX-A in muscle. In the case of excessive involuntary muscle contraction, such as with dystonia or spasticity, injecting the area of "most active EMG activity" may potentiate effects of botulinum toxin.[18,19]

For example, some clinicians probe within the small muscles of the forearm in a patient with focal dystonia to identify areas that seem to be the most "noisy" on EMG, and subsequently inject these areas. These audio signals are active motor unit potentials that sound like "rain on a tin roof" as opposed to the lower pitched seashell murmur of the motor endplate.

For patients with spasticity, the same scenario often exists. For example, the patient with a very tightly clenched fist (the "fisted hand") may have massive audio EMG discharges from the flexor digitorum sublimus muscle when the examiner attempts to passively stretch the fingers of the fisted hand. In this case, the author would

74

inject into the areas that are "noisiest" with EMG activity (as it would be impossible to localize the motor endplate with such excessive background noise.

Anatomic Method

Armed with the knowledge that motor endplates lie at the midpoint of muscle fibers, another injection method involves targeting the midpoint of muscle fibers based on an estimate of where the fibers are arranged within a muscle. This method is based on odds, the greater number of needle sticks and injection sites within a muscle, the more likely you are to infuse the toxin into the site of action within a muscle.

With only a few exceptions, the majority of motor endplates[15,20,21] will be found within the greatest bulk of a muscle. Exploiting this anatomic distribution, some clinicians identify the target muscle, draw a grid over the bulkiest portion of the muscle, and penetrate the skin at a number of the sites marked to distribute the toxin over a large area. This technique may be most useful in large, flat muscles like the trapezius, where motor point or endplate localization can be tedious.

Using careful measurements of the location of motor endplates in dog gastrocnemius muscles, the author compared the effectiveness of the anatomic method to the motor endplate targeting method.[5] The author's results were somewhat surprising, for in the small canine muscles significant differences comparing the two methods were found. The motor endplate targeting method was experimentally superior, and therefore the author recommends using EMG whenever possible.

While further research is needed to establish which method(s) are most desirable, treatment with BTX-A must always be individualized for the needs of the patient and the skills of the clinician.

SUGGESTED INJECTION SITES

In general, injection localization for BTX-A injection might best be decided using a hierarchy of findings. Consider injecting areas that manifest the following features, with more importance placed on findings at the top of the list:

1. **Areas of most active EMG motor unit firing (continuous noise of motor unit firing).** Finding continuously contracting motor units (the alpha motor neuron at its muscle fibers) when the patient is cooperative and voluntarily attempting to relax the muscle(s) of interest may be consistent with dystonia or alpha rigidity. When the clinician identifies these features, it may be best to inject the most active area of muscle regardless of whether or not a motor point or motor endplate can be identified.

2. **Motor endplates found in any muscle by EMG**

3. **Motor points in the following muscles:**
   Biceps, deltoid, flexor carp, radialis, flexor digitorum sublimus, vastus internus, sternomestoid, palmaris longus, tibialis anterior, and brachioradialis

4. **Myofascial trigger point(s) within the target muscle:** Since abnormal motor endplates are probably characteristic features of the trigger point,[7] it may be

76

desirable to inject these areas when found within the target muscle.

As there is considerable variation between investigators with regard to injection techniques, dosing and number of sites injected, the following section provides a general guide for a number of commonly treated muscles with botulinum toxin. However, every patient is different and circumstances may dictate variations in dosing and injection techniques. Therefore, treatment with BTX-A should always be individualized.

Information regarding available video and monograph on injection procedures found in Appendix A.

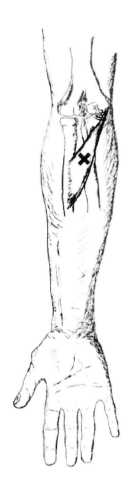

Figure 7-1: Suggested injection site for the **pronator teres muscle.**

78

Upper Limb

Pronator teres (facing page)

Action: pronates the wrist
Pitfalls: overweakening may cause difficulty with daily activities like opening jars
Injection location: corresponds to motor point.
BOTOX® Dose: 25-75 MU[22]
Dilution: 100MU in 1cc saline
Number of sites: 1

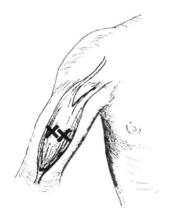

Figure 7-2. Suggested injection sites for **Biceps muscle**.

Action: flexes and supinates arm
Pitfalls: few
Injection location: corresponds to motor points
BOTOX® Dose: 100 MU[22]
Dilution: 100MU in 2cc saline
Number of sites: 2

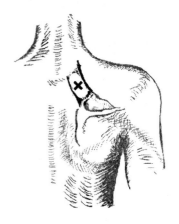

Figure 7-3. Suggested injection site for **Levator scapula muscle.**

Action: elevates scapula
Pitfalls: if too superficial, injection will be in trapezius; if too deep it will be in paraspinal muscle.
Injection location: As marked
BOTOX® dose: 50 MU
Dilution: 100MU in 1cc saline
Number of sites: 1

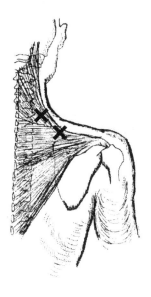

Figure 7-4. Suggested injection site for **Trapezius muscle**.

Action: many, depending on the portion of muscle contracting
Pitfalls: Unrealistic to expect to functionally weaken entire muscle. Select functional part of muscle (usually trigger points) such as upper aspect for injection rather than try to cover entire surface. Overlies many muscles of the thorax.
Injection location: As marked
BOTOX® dose: 10-15 MU/trigger point (50 MU total)

Lower limb

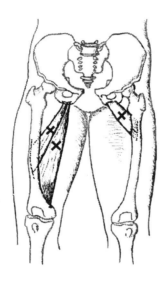

Figure 7-5. Suggested injection sites for **hip adductor muscles.**

Action: adduction of thigh
Pitfalls: (Using e-stim for localization): If electrical stimulation is too proximal, the needle may contact a branch of the obturator nerve rather than an intramuscular motor point.
Injection location: As marked
BOTOX® dose: 200MU/leg[22]
Dilution: 100MU in 3cc saline
Number of sites: 2-4/muscle

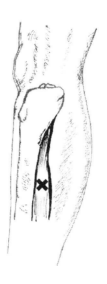

Figure 7-6. Suggest injection site for **Tibialis posterior muscle**.

Action: inverts and plantar flexes ankle
Pitfalls: difficult to localize with motor point stimulation; proximity to vessels in posterior compartment of lower limb.
Injection location: As marked
BOTOX® dose: 75MU[22]
Dilution: 100MU in 2cc saline
Number of sites: 1
Note: Author uses an anterior approach to this muscle

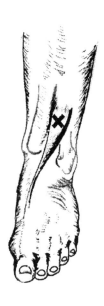

Figure 7-7. Suggested injection site for **Extensor hallicus longus muscle.**

Action: dorsiflexes great toe
Pitfalls: narrow window of needle insertion to hit muscle due to overlying fascia and tendons.
Injection location: As marked
BOTOX® dose: 50MU[22]
Dilution: 100MU in 1cc saline
Number of sites: 1

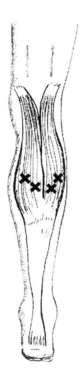

Figure 7-8. Suggested injected sites for **Gastrocnemius muscles.**

Action: ankle plantarflexion
Injection location: As marked
Pitfalls: motor point is proximal to endplate zone.
BOTOX® dose: 200MU[22]
Dilution: 100MU in 3cc saline
Number of sites: 2-4/each muscle

Back

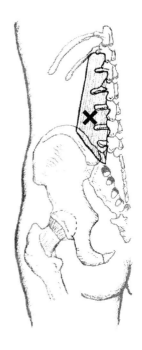

Figure 7-9. Suggested injection site for **Quadratus lumborum muscle.**

Action: lateral trunk flexor
Injection Location: As marked
Pitfalls: fluoroscopic, CT, or EMG guidance should be used.
BOTOX® dose: 100MU
Dilution: 100MU in 3cc saline
Number of sites: 1

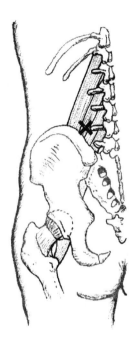

Figure 7-10. Suggested injection site for **Psoas muscle**.

Note: Injection depth can be gauged by aiming needle towards top of transverse process of L4 or L5, then redirect needle laterally into psoas.

Action: hip flexor
Injection Location: As marked
Pitfalls: fluoroscopic or CT guidance should be used.
BOTOX® dose: 200MU
Dilution: 100MU in 3cc saline
Number of sites: 1

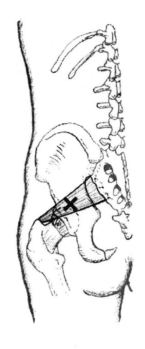

Figure 7-11. Suggested injection site for **Piriformis muscle**.

Action: external rotator of hip

Pitfalls: Fluoroscopy and/or EMG localization recommended. Injection too shallow will be in the gluteus maximus; too distal will be in gemelli or obturator internus.

Injection location: As marked.

BOTOX® dose: [23] 100MU

Dilution: 100MU in 3cc saline

Neck

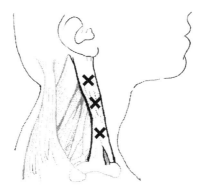

Figure 7-12. Suggested injection sites for **Sternocleidomastoid muscle**.

Action: contralateral neck rotation; anterior flexion
Pitfalls: proximity of muscle to vessels and pharynx
Injection location: As marked.
BOTOX® dose: 50MU
Dilution: 100MU in 1cc saline

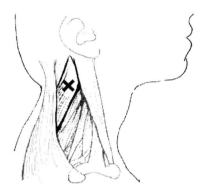

Figure 7-13. Suggested injection site for **Splenius capitus muscle**.

Action: ipsilateral rotation and extension of neck
Pitfalls: injection too posterior will be in trapezius; too anterior will be in SCM
Injection location: As marked.
BOTOX® dose: 50MU
Number of sites:1
Dilution: 100MU in 1cc saline

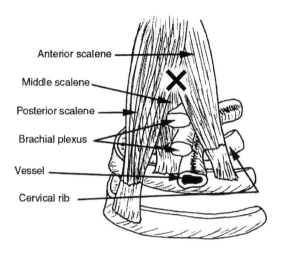

Anterior scalene
Middle scalene
Posterior scalene
Brachial plexus
Vessel
Cervical rib

Figure 7-14. Suggested injection site for **Scalene**[24] **muscles**.

Action: bends neck forward and laterally; raises 1st and 2nd ribs.
Pitfalls: proximity to vital structures; fluoroscopy and/or EMG recommended.
Injection location: As marked
BOTOX® dose: 35 MU
Dilution: 35MU in 1cc saline

REFERENCES

1. Bickerton LE, Agur AM, Ashby P. Flexor digitorum superficialis: locations of individual muscle bellies for botulinum toxin injections. Muscle Nerve 1997;20:1041-1043.

2. Borodic GE, Ferrante R, Pearce LB, Smith K. Histologic assessment of dose-related diffusion and muscle fiber response after therapeutic botulinum A toxin injections. Movement Disorders 1994;9:31-39.

3. Childers MK. Rationale for injection procedures for botulinum toxin type A in skeletal limb muscles. Eur J Neurol 1997;4(Suppl 2):37-40.

4. Shaari CM, Sanders I. Quantifying how location and dose of botulinum toxin injections affect muscle paralysis. Muscle Nerve 1993;16:964-969.

5. Childers MK, Kornegay JN, Aoki R, Otaviani L, Bogan DJ, Petroski G. Evaluating motor end-plate-targeted injections of botulinum toxin type A in a canine model. Muscle Nerve. 1998;21:653-655.

6. Hong CZ, Hsueh TC. Difference in pain relief after trigger point injections in myofascial pain patients with and without fibromyalgia [see comments]. Archives.of.Physical.Medicine & Rehabilitation. 1996;77:1161-1166.

7. Hong CZ, Simons DG. Pathophysiologic and electrophysiologic mechanisms of myofascial trigger points. [Review] [108 refs]. Archives.of.Physical.Medicine & Rehabilitation. 1998;79:863-872.

8. Awad EA. Muscle fiber and motor endplate [letter]. Arch Phys Med Rehabil. 1980;61:149-149.

9. Awad EA, Awad OE. Injection techniques for spasticity. Minneapolis, MN: E.A. Awad,M.D.,P.A.; 1993.

10. Wiederholt WC. "End-plate noise" in electromyography. Neurology. 1970;20:214-224.

11. Brown WF, Varkey GP. The origin of spontaneous electrical activity at the end-plate zone. Ann Neurol. 1981;10:557-560.

12. Buchthal F. Spontaneous electrical activity: an overview. [Review]. Muscle Nerve. 1982;5:S52-S59

13. Halpern D, Meelhuysen FE. Phenol motor point block in the management of muscular hypertonia. Arch Phys Med Rehabil. 1966;47:659-664.

14. Halpern D. Histologic studies in animals after intramuscular neurolysis with phenol. Arch Phys Med Rehabil. 1977;58:438-443.

15. Coers C. The innervation of muscle. Springfield,IL: Charles Thomas; 1959.

16. Hesse S, Jahnke MT, Luecke D, Mauritz KH. Short-term electrical stimulation enhances the effectiveness of Botulinum toxin in the treatment of lower limb spasticity in hemiparetic patients. Neuroscience Letters 1995;201:37-40.

17. Rosales RL, Arimura K, Takenaga S, Osame M. Extrafusal and intrafusal muscle effects in experimental botulinum toxin-A

injection. Muscle Nerve 1996;19:488-496.

18. Brans JW, de Boer IP, Aramideh M, Ongerboer de Visser BW, Speelman JD. Botulinum toxin in cervical dystonia: low dosage with electromyographic guidance. J Neurol. 1995;242:529-534.

19. Speelman JD, Brans JW. Cervical dystonia and botulinum treatment: is electromyographic guidance necessary? Movement Disorders. 1995;10:802-802.

20. Coers C. Structural organization of the motor nerve endings in mammalian muscle spindles and other striated muscle fibers. Am J Phys Med Rehabil. 1958;38:166-175.

21. Coers C. The vital staining of muscle biopsies with methylene blue. J Neurol Neurosurg Psychiatry. 1952;15:211

22. Brin MF. Dosing, administration, and a treatment algorithm for use of botulinum toxin A for adult-onset spasticity. In: Brin MF, ed. Spasticity: etiology, evaluation, management, and the role of botulinum toxin type A. John Wiley & Sons; 1997:S208-S220

23. Galate JF, Childers MK, Gnatz S. Effectiveness of botulinum toxin in refractory piriformis muscle syndrome. Arch Phys Med Rehabil. 1997;78:1041(Abstract)

24. Monsivais JJ, Monsivais DB. Botulinum toxin in painful syndromes. Hand Clinics. 1996;12:787-789.

8

CHAPTER

Co-author: Daniel J Wilson, PhD

Documentation

Important items to document when treating patients for painful muscular syndromes with botulinum toxin type A are previous treatment, response to prior treatment, medical work-up, plan for future treatment and measures of response to treatment planned.

Measuring musculoskeletal pain is a complex issue due to the nature of individual recognition and interpretation of pain. The complexity of evaluating pain intensity lead Melzack and colleagues to formulate the gate control theory of pain.[1] This conceptual model of pain perception was expanded from a pure sensory model to a model encompassing sensory, motivational and cognitive components. Despite an expanded understanding of the psychological basis of pain intensity, the relationship between pain and musculoskeletal pathophysiology remains in need of instruments that measure self-report and physical function.

Experts[2;3] have proposed criteria for ideal assessment methods that incorporate reliable, sensitive ratio scales that separately assess sensory and affective dimensions of pain. The ideal method would include data about the accuracy and reliability of patients. Some examples of self-report scales developed to estimate pain intensity using these criteria are the Verbal Rating Scale, the Visual Analog Scale, and the Numerical Rating Scale. Each of these scales was designed to measure pain intensity and provide statistical data. However, these instruments do not provide information about musculoskeletal limitations imposed by pain.

Evaluating Effects Of Pain on Physical Function

Assessment of range-of-motion, using a "two inclinometer" technique is an example of a test used to evaluate the physical effects/limitations imposed by pain is.[4] These and examples of other tests used to evaluate the physical effects/limitations imposed by pain are summarized in Table 1. While these instruments are physiologically relevant, they do not provide information about the intensity of pain perceived by the patient.

Table 1. Physical capacity tests used to evaluate the effects of musculoskeletal pain and their statistical properties.

<u>**Range of Motion**</u>
      Two inclinometer test
      Valid relative to lumbar flexion and extension [5]
      Intra- and intertester reliability established [6].
<u>**Trunk Strength**</u>
      Cybex® Isokinetic Device
      Proven validity and repeatability [7;8]
<u>**Lifting Capacity**</u>
      Cybex® Liftask
      Comparative norms established [9]

A sample BTX-A injection template follows:

Pre-procedure dx: _____
Post-procedure dx: _____

Examples: (ICD 9 Code after each)
Spasmotic torticollis _____
Spastic hemiplegia _____
Etc. _____

Response to prior treatment:
Patient global assessment score: _____

Current level of function:
Patient global assessment score: _____
Analogue pain score: _____
Physician global assessment score: _____

Exam: Example of specific exams for dystonia, or spasticity:

Ashworth score (for spasticity):
_____ fingers ___wrist ____elbow ____shoulder
_____ ankle ____knee ___hip

Tsui Torticollis Rating Scale (for cervical dystonia)
A. Amplitude of sustained movements (0-9):
Rotation (0=absent, 1=<15°, 2=15-30°, 3=>30°)
Tilt (0-absent, 1=<15°, 2=15-30°, 3=>30°)
Ante/retro (0=absent,mild,2=moderate,3=severe)
Combined = score Ax B
B. Duration of sustained movements (0-2):

1 = intermittent, 2 = constant
C. Shoulder elevation (0-3): 0=absent, 1=mild & intermittent, 2=mild & constant, or severe and intermittent, 3=severe and constant
D. Head tremor (0-4):
Severity (1=mild, 2=severe)
Duration (1=occasional, 2=continuous)
Severity x duration = score D

Total torticollis score = [A x B] + C + D (0-25) = _____

If EMG is used: EMG:
(95860-26)

A limited needle EMG was performed in muscles of the (upper/lower ext; neck) to assess for involuntary contractions, which were identified in the following muscles:

___FDS Flexor digitorum sublimis
___FDL Flexor digitorum longus
___SCM Sternocleidomastoid
___FDP Flexor digitorum profundus
___EHL Extensor hallucis longus
___SC   Splenius capitis
___FCR Flexor carpi radialis
___Ptib   Posterior tibialis
___Trap Trapezius
___FCU Flexor carpi ulnaris
___Gastr Gastrocnemius
___PL Pollicis longus
___Biceps
___Other:_____

Procedure: The skin overlying each target muscle was prepared with alcohol and thoroughly cleaned. Under clean conditions, a 25 gauge 50mm dual port injection needle/EMG electrode was introduced into each muscle belly under continuous EMG guidance. Prior to injection, the syringe was withdrawn to insure that vascular structures were not penetrated, and a continuous EMG signal was monitored during injection. The following muscles were injected with BTX-A, reconstituted to a dilution of 100MU/1cc preservative free saline:

Consent

Following EMG exam and interpretation of findings, and prior to procedures, consent should be obtained from the patient for treatment with botulinum toxin. The risks, benefits and alternative treatments should be explained and time allowed for patient questions.

A sample consent form is included in Appendix B.

REFERENCES

1. Melzack R, Wall PD. Pain mechanisms: a new theory. [Review] [77 refs]. *Science.* 1965;150:971-979.
2. Price DD, Harkins SW. Psychophysical approaches to pain measurement and assessment. In: Turk DC, Melzak R, eds. *Handbook of pain assessment.* New York: The Guilford Press; 1992:111-134.
3. Gracely RH, Dubner R. Pain assessment in humans -- a reply to Hall. *Pain.* 1981;11:109-120.
4. Engelberg A. *American Medical Association guides to the evaluation of permanent impairment.* Chicago: American Medical Association; 1988.
5. Mayer T, Kishino N, Keeley J, Mayer H, Mooney V. Using physical measures to assess low back pain. *J musculoskeletal med.* 1985;6:44-59.
6. Keeley J, Mayer TG, Cox R, Gatchel RJ, Smith J, Mooney V. Quantification of lumbar function. Part 5: Reliability of range- of-motion measures in the sagittal plane and an in vivo torso rotation measurement technique. *Spine.* 1986;11:31-35.
7. Langrana NA, Lee CK. Isokinetic evaluation of trunk muscles. *Spine.* 1984;9:171-175.
8. Smith SS, Mayer TG, Gatchel RJ, Becker TJ. Quantification of lumbar function. Part 1: Isometric and multispeed isokinetic trunk strength

measures in sagittal and axial planes in normal subjects. *Spine.* 1985;10:757-764.

9. Mayer T, Gatchel R, Keeley J, Mayer H, Richland D. Building industrial databases:Physical capacity measurements specific to major job categories in U.S. railroads. *Proc int soc.* 1991

9
CHAPTER

Author: Diane Simison, PhD

Obtaining Reimbursement

The current coverage and reimbursement by third party payers for botulinum toxin has been developed for botulinum toxin type A (BOTOX®), since BOTOX® is the only botulinum toxin approved by the US FDA at this time. Therefore, the information in this chapter is specific to BOTOX® coverage and reimbursement policies. As other botulinum toxins enter the market, each may have slightly different coverage policies and reimbursement mechanisms based on specific approved labeling, clinical characteristics and formulations. Most major third-party payers will provide coverage and reimbursement for botulinum toxin type A. However, obtaining reimbursement will require your attention.

- The rules and requirements for obtaining coverage and reimbursement will vary by payer.
- Reimbursement amounts will be different for each payer.
- Reimbursement rules and amounts can vary for each setting of care (such as: physician's office, hospital outpatient clinic, ambulatory surgery center).

This chapter includes important information on the coverage and reimbursement for botulinum toxin type A treatment by third-party payers. The chapter includes:

- A general overview of payer policies on coverage and reimbursement for BTX-A treatment
- Important considerations in preparing claims
- Additional information specific to coverage and reimbursement in various treatment settings

To obtain reimbursement from a third-party payer, your patient must have an insurance benefit that will include coverage for BTX-A treatment. You should verify the patient's benefits and obtain instructions from the payer for filing the reimbursement claim. Precise instructions can be obtained from the patient's insurance company.

A REVIEW OF THIRD-PARTY PAYER REQUIREMENTS

In this section, the important aspects of obtaining coverage and reimbursement for BTX-A treatment from third-party payers are reviewed. Since Medicare has the most specific requirements, the discussion for this payer is more detailed.

Medicare: Insurer of those over age 65 and the disabled

Since BTX-A treatment will be administered in the outpatient setting, it will fall under Part B of the Medicare Part B benefit. About 20 different Medicare carriers administer the Medicare outpatient benefit and process claims for 56 states or state regions. A separate policy or guideline has been issued by Medicare carriers for coverage and reimbursement for BTX-A treatment for each state or state region.

- BTX-A treatment will be reimbursed when

administered by a physician to a Medicare-eligible patient

- Regional Medicare Carriers have some latitude in determining coverage policies; therefore there is some variability in the coverage for BTX-A treatment used with pain diagnoses under Medicare
- Reimbursement will be triggered by the presence of approved CPT procedure codes and ICD-9 diagnosis codes on the HCFA 1500 claim form; prior authorization is not required
- BTX-A treatment will be reimbursed when administered in various outpatient settings, including the physician's office, hospital outpatient clinics, and ambulatory surgery centers, including pain clinics, but not for all diagnoses and procedures
- BTX-A should be billed using code J0585 (botulinum toxin type A, per unit)
- Reimbursement for BTX-A treatment will be 80 percent of the allowable amount; the patient pays the other 20 percent
- The Medicare allowable amount for BTX-A treatment currently is 95 percent of the average wholesale price of the drug (AWP)

**Diagnosis And Procedure Codes Are Important
To Reimbursement**

Medicare will reimburse the cost of BTX-A treatment when it is used with a covered ("payable") diagnosis. Covered diagnoses will be listed in the local coverage policies issued by the Medicare Carriers. If BTX-A treatment is medically necessary for a diagnosis not listed as covered, you should submit documentation supporting the medical necessity and clinical literature [1-4] supporting the use to the Carrier.

103

As with ICD-9 diagnosis codes, Medicare policies list the CPT procedure codes for which BTX-A treatment will be reimbursed. Medicare does not currently list CPT code 20550 as covered in policies for BTX-A treatment.

A list of codes that might be used for pain indications is shown in Table 1.

Coverage guidelines - ICD-9 and CPT Code Pairings

In many cases, Medicare provides guidelines for coverage of BTX-A treatment. For Medicare, a coverage guideline consists of a CPT code that is payable when used with specified ICD-9 diagnosis. If a Medicare Carrier has implemented coverage guidelines, the paired codes are listed in the Medicare policy for each state.

Electromyography Procedure Coding

Medicare will pay for electromyography when used in association with a BTX-A injection. Medicare policies list covered electromyography codes. Those most frequently covered appear in Table 1.

CPT code 95870 (electromyography, other than paraspinal e.g., abdomen, thorax) was listed as a new code in 1998, and for that reason is not yet included in most Medicare policies for BTX-A treatment. Therefore, when using this code, medical necessity should be documented and submitted to the Carrier, together with support from the clinical literature.

Proper Use Of Modifiers Is Essential to Medicare Reimbursement

Modifiers document specific information regarding the procedure, such as the anatomic area of the body being treated (anatomical) or aspects of the procedure itself that have been altered (procedural). Modifiers are to be recorded on the claim form.

In the case of Medicare, correct use of modifiers can be associated with higher reimbursement rates, and incorrect use can be associated with claims denials or "downcoding" (where a lesser amount of reimbursement is paid).

Medicare Policies Contain Instructions on Dosage And Number of Injections

Medicare policies may include limits on the amount of a drug that is to be used for types of muscles, or the number of injections that may be reimbursed per site. Medicare defines a "site" as noncontiguous muscle groups. Only one injection will be reimbursed per site.

The dosage limits may specify the amount of the drug that is reimbursable for muscles of various sizes, or the number of injections that are may be reimbursable over a certain period of time.

You should obtain the payer's written policy regarding limitations on dosage or number of injections of botulinum toxin, and follow the coding instructions accordingly.

Medicare Will Pay for Discarded Botulinum Toxin Type A under Certain Conditions

Medicare Carriers will pay for BTX-A that must be discarded, and has established certain rules for how the wastage is to be recorded. You should obtain a copy of the payer's written instructions, and then follow the payer rules concerning how the discarded amount is to be billed and documented in the patient's medical record.

Medicare Requires Documentation

Medicare requires that the medical necessity for a procedure be documented in the patient's record. Occasionally, a payer will require the submission of a letter of medical necessity prior to approval of payment.

In these cases, you should submit a letter of medical necessity for treatment with BTX-A to the insurance plan medical director. Your letter should include the following information:

- Reason for treatment
- Physical examination findings
- Impression, including primary and secondary diagnosis and their effects
- Prior treatments
- Plan and recommendations, including why BTX-A treatment is being prescribed, injection areas
- Conclusion, including diagnosis codes, dosage, areas of injection, follow-up needed

MEDICAID

Medicaid is a joint federal and state entitlement program providing health care benefits for low income individuals who are aged, disabled or blind. The coverage amount of reimbursement, as well as how BTX-A treatment must be obtained, will vary among the states.

- Regardless of the treatment setting, BTX-A treatment will usually be covered under the Physician Services Program; in some cases, it may be covered under the Outpatient Prescription Drug Program
- Physicians will be reimbursed for BTX-A based on the average wholesale price (AWP) minus a percentage (usually about 10 percent); reimbursement for other procedures is provided in a variety of ways, such as by fee schedule, actual cost or an approved charge
- Prior approval of BTX-A treatment may be necessary

In some states, BTX-A must be billed and paid under the patient's Medicaid outpatient pharmacy drug benefit. You must check with your state Medicaid office to determine if this is required in your state. If it is required, the patient must pick up BTX-A at a Medicaid-approved pharmacy and bring it to the physician's office for injection. The pharmacy will bill Medicaid for the BTX-A.

COMMERCIAL AND MANAGED CARE INSURERS

Commercial and managed care payers will cover BTX-A treatment for FDA-approved uses and for some other uses as well when medically necessary and when the use is supported in the clinical literature.

Many commercial insurers have adopted the principles of managed care, where the patient must see a physician in the payer network and treatment may be restricted by a treatment guideline. In all cases, the insurance plan requirements must be determined prior to treatment with botulinum toxin.

- Coverage and reimbursement will vary based on the provisions of the patient's insurance plan and the setting in which BTX-A is administered
- Prior authorization, or pre-certification, of the use of BTX-A will be necessary in many cases
- Documentation of medical necessity will be required for prior authorization
- Coverage for BTX-A treatment may depend on the plan formulary
- The insurer's medical director often decides coverage for expensive pharmaceuticals, after reviewing other treatment options and the medical necessity.

If a treatment is given before required prior authorization is obtained, the payer may deny coverage and the patient may be required to pay the cost of botulinum toxin. Therefore, it should be determined before treatment if prior authorization will be required. A call may be made to the patient's insurance plan to obtain this information.

WORKERS' COMPENSATION

Each state has a program to pay for treatment of workers injured during job performance. The requirements and characteristics of each state program are different, but there are some similarities.

- Return to work is the goal for all workers' compensation programs
- All necessary health care is paid for if it is medically necessary

- Some states will require pre-certification for treatments with BTX-A
- Most states reimburse for medical services based on fee schedules
- Some states have treatment guidelines, where therapy must be listed prior to coverage

Some workers' compensation programs have established treatment guidelines and have referenced treatment with botulinum toxin. For example, BTX-A is referenced in the lower extremity treatment guideline adopted by workers' compensation in Texas. You can obtain this information from each state workers' compensation agency.

COVERAGE AND BILLING FOR BOTULINUM TOXIN TYPE A TREATMENT; MECHANISMS OF PAYMENT

The requirements and the process for obtaining payment for BTX-A treatment will vary by the payer and the setting of care in which treatment is delivered.

Payers recognize whether a claim is payable and enforce payment restrictions through review of the claim for reimbursement that is submitted. Those components of the claim that are important to obtaining payment for BTX-A treatment are reviewed below.

IMPORTANT ISSUES FOR TYPE A TREATMENT USED TO TREAT PAIN

Trigger Point Injections

You should determine whether you are treating the trigger point or whether you are treating the surrounding spasm.

You must examine your coding options prior to selecting a code that best represents the nature of the treatment.

To date, no Medicare carrier policy list CPT codes 20550 (injection, tendon sheath, ligament, trigger point) or diagnosis 729.1 as covered codes for BTX-A injections.

Special Payer Rules for the Pain Clinic

Reimbursement of the Ambulatory Surgery Center by Medicare

If you are administering treatment with BTX-A in a pain clinic rather than your office, the clinic must be classified as a place of service on the HCFA 1500 claim form. This code provides the appropriate coverage and reimbursement information for the services rendered.

Most pain clinics will be classified as ambulatory surgery center (ASC), a hospital outpatient department or an outpatient rehabilitation clinic. Only you can determine which classification is correct. The facility and the physician will both receive payments for treatment in these settings.

Ambulatory surgery centers are paid prospectively. If the treatment is one approved by Medicare to be given in an ambulatory surgery center, the CPT procedure is grouped into one of eight ASC payment groups. The group assignment determines the amount that Medicare pays for facility services furnished in connection with a covered procedure. There is no separate payment for BTX-A furnished by the facility. Your fee as a physician will be billed in addition to the ASC payment.

If the CPT procedure is grouped into an ASC payment but delivered in a hospital outpatient department instead of an ambulatory surgery center, the facility payment is the lesser of a blended rate (42 percent of the hospital's reasonable costs or charges and 58 percent of the ASC payment rate). Pharmaceuticals used in ASC-approved procedures performed in the hospital outpatient department are generally covered separately, and charges for them are used in the calculation of the payment rate.

HOW TO OBTAIN INFORMATION ABOUT COVERAGE AND PAYMENT FOR BOTULINUM TOXIN TYPE A TREATMENT

There are sources for information about coverage and reimbursement for BTX-A used to treat pain.

• **Your Medicare Part B Carrier**
You can obtain the policy detailing requirements for obtaining reimbursement for BTX-A treatment from your Medicare Part B Carrier. If you do not have the name and address of the Carrier, you can locate it on the HCFA website at http://www.hcfa.gov.

• **Your patient's insurance company**
The patient's insurance company will verify the patient's benefit so that you can be sure that reimbursement will be forthcoming. The insurance company will also be able to tell you if pre-certification is required, other requirements for submitting claims, and what the reimbursement amount will be.

REFERENCES

1. Childers MK, Kornegay JN, Aoki R, Otaviani L, Bogan DJ, Petroski G. Evaluating motor end-plate-targeted injections of botulinum toxin type A

111

in a canine model. Muscle Nerve. 1998;21:653-655.
2. Shaari CM, Sanders I. Quantifying how location and dose of botulinum toxin injections affect muscle paralysis. Muscle Nerve 1993;16:964-969.
3. Childers MK. Rationale for injection procedures for botulinum toxin type A in skeletal limb muscles. Eur J Neurol 1997;4(Suppl 2):37-40.
4. Bickerton LE, Agur AM, Ashby P. Flexor digitorum superficialis: locations of individual muscle bellies for botulinum toxin injections. Muscle Nerve 1997;20:1041-1043.

Table 1. Pain-Related CPT and ICD-9 Codes Approved by Most Medicare Part B Carriers

ICD-9 Diagnosis Codes
- 728.85 - other disorders of muscle, ligament, fascia, spasm of muscle
- 333-333.9 - dystonias
- 342-342.1 - hemiplegia and hemiparesis
- 343-343.9 - cerebral palsy

CPT Procedure Codes
- 64640 - destruction by neurolytic agent; other peripheral nerve or branch
- 64612 - destruction by neurolytic agent; muscles enervated by facial nerve
- 64613 - destruction by neurolytic agent; cervical spinal muscles

Coding Guideline
- 728.85 with 64640

Electromyography
- 95860 - needle electromyography, one extremity
- 95867 - needle electromyography, cranial nerve supplied muscles, unilateral
- 95868 - needle electromyography, cranial nerve supplied muscles, bilateral
- 95869 - needle electromyography, limited study of specific muscles (to be replaced with code 95870)
- 95870 - needle electromyography, other than paraspinal muscles

113

Appendix A:

Additional Sources of Information

1. Portable, audio EMG units
2. Stimulators
3. Video/ monograph information
4. Injection training seminars/workshops
5. Author contact information

1. Portable Audio EMG Units

Portable audio EMG
Allergan BOTOX® EMG Amplifier
Allergan Customer Service Department
1-800-377-7790

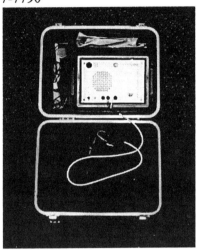

Price: Aprox. $750 (US)

2. Portable nerve stimulators/TENS:

Nerve stimulators and pain management instruments:
Life Tech, Inc.
http://www.life-tech.com

2 channel Tens unit:
Intelect®Tens unit $79.00
Rallis corp.
1-800-852-8898
http://www.rallis.com

3. Video and Monograph Information

"Emerging treatment options for myofascial pain syndromes"
Discovery International
520 Lake Cook Road, Suite 250
Deerfield, IL 60015 USA
1-847-374-4600 (voice)
1-847-374-4650 (fax)
http://www.discovery-intl.com

4. Injection training workshops/seminars

Society for Pain Practice Management
11111 Nall #202
Leawood, KS 66211 USA
1-913-491-6451 (voice)
1-913-491-6453 (fax)
http://www.sppm.org

Dannemiller Memorial Educational Foundation
12500 Network Boulevard, Suite 101
San Antonio, TX 78249-3302 USA
1-800-328-2308 (voice)
1-210-641-8329 (fax)
http://www.pain.com

WE MOVE – Worldwide Education and
Awareness for Movement Disorders
Mount Sinai Medical Center
One Gustave L. Levy Place Box 1052
New York, NY 10029 USA
1-800-437-MOV2 (voice)
1-212-987-7363 (fax)
http://www.wemove.org

116

American Academy of Physical Medicine and
Rehabilitation (AAPM&R)
One IBM Plaza, Suite 2500
Chicago, IL 60611-3604 USA
1-312-464-9700 (voice)
1-312-464-0227 (fax)
http://www.aapmr.org

5.   Authors may be contacted at the following addresses:

Martin K. Childers, D.O.
Assistant Professor
Department of Physical Medicine and Rehabilitation
University of Missouri-Columbia
Columbia, MO 65212 USA
Email: childersmk@health.missouri.edu

Daniel J. Wilson, PhD
Assistant Professor
Department of Physical Medicine and Rehabilitation
University of Missouri-Columbia
Columbia, MO 65212 USA

Diane Simison, PhD
Principal
Epinomics Research, Inc
2320 N. Tuckahoe Street,
Arlington, VA 22205 USA

Appendix B:

1.   **Sample Consent Form**

BOTULINUM TOXIN TYPE A INJECTION FOR TREATMENT OF DYSTONIA, SPASTICITY, OR PAINFUL SYNDROMES

Dystonia is a neurologic disorder manifested by involuntary, sustained contractions (spasms) of muscles producing abnormal postures. Injections of botulinum toxin type A (BOTOX®), a protein that causes temporary weakness of the injected muscles, may provide effective relief for dystonia, hemifacial spasm (involuntary twitching of one side of the face), spasticity and other painful conditions due to involuntary muscle contractions. Studies involving many patients have demonstrated the safety and effectiveness of this form of treatment.

Botulinum toxin type A, though approved by the FDA for treatment of blepharospasm and hemifacial spasm, has not been approved in treating dystonias, spasticity, or muscle pain. However, the American Academy of Neurology has deemed this drug safe and effective in the treatment of oromandibular, cervical, spasmodic, and focal dystonia. In addition, the National Institute of Health has also issued a consensus statement that this drug is effective and safe in treating these disorders.

In addition to dystonia, recent clinical reports in the medical literature indicate that botulinum toxin type A treatments are safe and effective in the treatment of muscle spasticity (involuntary spasms often seen after spinal cord injury, head injury, and other neurologic disorders). Patients that have had head injuries and strokes often have symptoms with elements of both spasticity and

119

dystonia.

An alternative to botulinum toxin type A therapy would be medications taken by mouth such as diazepam, benztropine, clonazepam, baclofen, and others. Additionally, certain physical therapies are known to be beneficial in the disorder as well.

You may be videotaped prior to and while receiving the medication. By signing this consent form, you give your permission to have Dr.   or his assistants, make photographs, videotapes, and/or recordings of these injections, under the condition that these photographs, etc., will be used in the interest of medical teaching, research, or health science. These photographs, tapes or recordings and information relating to your case may be published and republished in professional journals or medical books.

The procedure will consist of the following: You will receive the botulinum toxin type A by injection into the muscle through the skin. The skin will be cleaned with an alcohol pad, and the site to be injected may be determined by using a small electric stimulator that is connected to a battery or a larger machine that is called an EMG machine. This allows the physician to correctly localize the proper area of the muscle to inject. A small electric current may applied onto the surface of the skin or just beneath the surface of the skin with a small, sterilized needle. You will usually receive three needle sticks to each muscle for even distribution of the drug, and approximately 0.3 ccs of fluid (less than a teaspoon) will be injected with each needle insertion.

Botulinum toxin type A may relieve symptoms for three to six months. You may notice some improvement within the next 72 hours but may not notice anything for up to two weeks. If at any time you are uncomfortable during the procedure, please let us know.

Potential benefits of this treatment would include reduction in painful spasms, increased ability to range a joint such as the ankle, knee, or arm, potential to increase the speed of walking and other functional abilities, and potential for certain physical therapies to be performed more easily, such as splinting and casting.

There are risks involved in botulinum toxin type A injections. Common side effects include muscle weakness that may affect function of the limb treated, local bruising, and discomfort at the injection site. There are other conditions listed below in which these injections are performed. The common side effects related to the following disorders and their treatment include:

For treatment of Blepharospasm (involuntary eye closing):
      ptosis (eyelid drooping)
      diplopia (double vision)
      burning and pain
      eyelid swelling and bruising
      tearing

For treatment of Oromandibular dystonia:

121

dysphasia (swallowing and chewing difficulties)
dysarthria (talking difficulty)
hoarseness
drooling

For treatment of Cervical dystonia:
dysphasia
dysarthria
singing difficulty
neck weakness

For treatment of Hemifacial spasm:
facial weakness

For treatment of Focal dystonia:
hand weakness and foot drop

Rare side effects have been reported but are not necessarily a result of the botulinum toxin. These include:
nausea
muscle sorenessheadaches
light-headedness
fever
chills
hypertension
weakness
difficulty breathing
diarrhea
abdominal pain

Special Warning of Risk to Females of Childbearing Potential

The effects of botulinum toxin type A on human babies are unknown, but could cause harm. For this reason it is necessary to:
1. Use adequate birth control to avoid getting pregnant while receiving treatment.
2. Inform me immediately if you get pregnant.

This treatment may cause an allergic reaction. Potentially, this reaction could be severe and life threatening.

As is true of all medications in medical treatment, there is always the possibility of a new or unexpected risk.

For the reasons stated above, if you have any worrisome symptoms please notify me immediately. My telephone number is. _____

By signing this consent form, I acknowledge that I have read and understand this information and that Dr _____ _____ has explained the potential risks and benefits of this procedure to me. Additionally, there has been adequate time allowed for me to ask questions, and Dr._ _____ has responded to my satisfaction.

_____   _____   _____
Signature of Patient   Witness   Date

When the patient is a minor or incompetent to give consent:

I, _____hereby certify that I am ____
_____(relationship to patient)of _____
_____ and am duly authorized to execute
the foregoing.(name of patient) _____

_____

_____ _____ _____
Signature   Witness   Date

Index

1a afferents, 50
acetylcholine, 4, 9-13, 15,
    17-   19, 35, 68
    physiology of, 9
action potential, 10-12, 15
alpha rigidity, 15, 18, 75
anesthetic agents, 35,36
antispastic agents, 56, 58
    GABA, 56
ATP, 16, 18, 20
Atracurium, 12, 35, 36
Beatty's maneuver, 39, 40
BOTOX®, 1, 2, 77-90, 98,
    111
botulinum toxin type A
    ceiling dose, 5
    dystonia and, 2, 15,
        25, 26, 55, 58
    licensed treatments,
        2
    median lethal
        dose, 4
    myofascial pain
        and, 2, 22, 23, 31,
        35-   38
    published uses, 2
    relative
        contraindications,
        7
    side effects, 12, 14,
        117, 118
    spasticity and, 2,
        15, 17, 22, 24,
        26, 27
celiac plexus, 13
clonidine, 57
consent form, 115
dantrolene sodium, 57
disability scores, 37

disordered motor control, 50
documentation
    BTX-A injection
    template, 95
    consent, 11
Dunteman, Ed MD, 36
dystonia, 2, 15, 25, 26, 55,
    58
    afferent nerves and,
        61
    definition of, 58
    off painful
        dystonia, 26
    pain and, 22, 24-26
    symptoms of, 55,
        59
Dystonia Medical Research
    Foundation, 60
electrical stimulation (estim),
    73, 93
electromyography (EMG),
    18, 34, 40, 42, 60, 64, 68,
    101, 109
endplate potential, 10, 18
endplate zones, 27, 67, 69,
    84
excessive salivation, 14, 17
FDA, 1, 2, 98, 104, 115
fluoroscopy, 7, 65, 87, 90
focal dystonia, 22, 25, 59, 60,
    73, 115, 118
gamma motor neuron, 51, 55
gastroc-soleus, 16
gate control theory of pain,
    93
global assessment, 37
glycolysis, 16, 18
H reflex, 40, 54
hyperhydrosis, 2, 14, 17

125

inhibitory casting, 54
injection locations
        anatomic method,
    68, 73, 74
        motor endplates,
    34, 66-70, 73-75

EMG activity method, 73
involuntary muscle
    contraction, 15, 22, 35, 59,
    60, 73, 115
loss of sensation, 36, 42
mechanoreceptors, 50
median nerve compression,
    42
motor endplates, 34, 66-70,
    73-35
muscle
        extrafusal, 50, 57
        intrafusal, 50
        skeletal, 9-11, 17-
    20, 50, 51, 66
        smooth, 10, 11, 13,
    19-21
        Type I, 16, 20
        Type II, 16, 18
muscle fibers, 16, 18, 30, 32,
    50, 53, 57, 67, 69, 70, 73,
    74
muscle spasms, 52, 56, 58
muscle spindles, 50, 53,
muscular hyperactivity, 27,
    56
muscular weakness, 5, 7
myofascial pain syndrome, 2,
    30, 31, 35, 37, 38
myoglobin, 16
myosin, 11
nerve conduction test, 40
nerve fibers, 4, 35
neuromuscular junction, 9,
    18, 19, 67
neurotransmitter, 9, 12, 13,

17-20
nitric oxide, 10, 19
numerical rating scale, 94
off painful dystonia (OPD),
    26
oxidative phosphorylation,
    16, 18, 20
pain, 4, 5, 12, 13, 22-27, 33
phenol neurolysis, 15
piriformis syndrome, 27, 40,
    41
postganglionic, 13, 14, 20
postganglionic sympathetic
    neuron, 12, 13, 19
preganglionic
parasympathetic   neuron, 11,
    12, 19
pressure algometer reading,
    37
pronator teres syndrome, 38,
    41-43, 46
receptors
        ionotropic, 9, 12,
    18
        muscarinic, 10, 11,
    13, 19, 20
        nicotinic, 9, 11, 12,
    17-20
referred pain, 32, 33
reimbursement
        ambulatory surgery
    centers and, 98, 107
        commercial
    insurance, 104
        coverage
guidelines, 101, 104
        diagnosis codes,
    100, 103, 109
        EMG coding, 101,
    109
        managed care, 104
insurance mechanisms of
payment

---

*Academic Information
Systems*